Contents

Management of Respiratory Insufficiency

Respiratory insufficiency can arise from a variety of etiologies and discussion of specific etiologies is beyond the scope of this pocket guide. However, respiratory insufficiency generally falls into the following categories: hypoxemia, hypercarbia, inability to maintain a secure and effective airway, or a combination of all these problems.

Patients who are unable to maintain a patent and a secure airway such as patients with depressed mental status or patients with significant narrowing of the airway (extrinsic = compression from outside, or intrinsic = narrowing from inside) generally will need their trachea intubated and they often then need to be assisted with mechanical ventilation. These patients generally do not have hypoxemia, but may have hypercarbia due to hypoventilation or airway obstruction.

Patients with hypoxemic respiratory failure will need oxygen supplementation. Oxygen may be administered by various respiratory devices (discussed below) depending on the degree of hypoxemia and (consequently) the concentrations of oxygen necessary to attain and maintain satisfactory hemoglobin oxygen saturation between 88 – 93%.

In general, one proceeds from devices that deliver lower concentrations of oxygen (21 – 35%) to devices that deliver modest concentrations of oxygen (35-60%) to devices that are capable of delivering high concentrations of oxygen (80-100%). We will discuss each of these devices below:

a. Nasal Cannula:

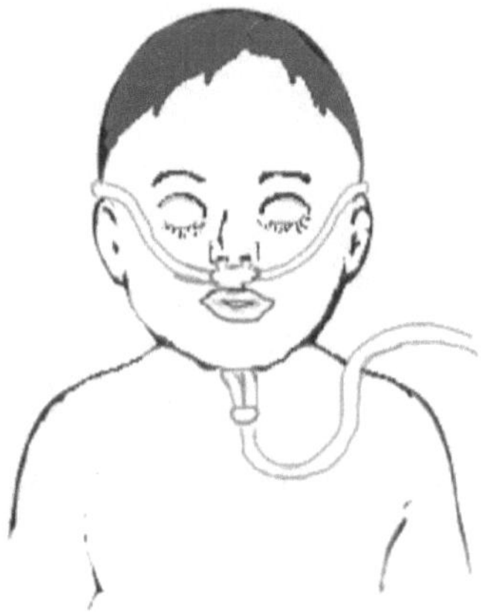

A nasal cannula consists of two soft nasal prongs of various sizes (from infants to adult sizes) that fit into the patient's nostrils. These prongs are attached to long tubing that is connected to the oxygen source. The tubing is usually looped around patient's ears and secured with a tape to the patient's cheeks. The flow of oxygen determines **the approximate concentration of oxygen** that is delivered to the patient as follows:

1 liter/min oxygen flow	⟶	24% oxygen
2 liters/min oxygen flow	⟶	28% oxygen
3 liters/min oxygen flow	⟶	32% oxygen
4 liters/min oxygen flow	⟶	36% oxygen

It is important to recognize that these are approximate concentrations. With higher flow rates of oxygen it is difficult to be certain exactly what the actual concentration of oxygen the patient is receiving. Changes in the rate and depth of respiration, and the degree of mouth breathing are factors that alter the room air entrainment resulting in variations in the oxygen concentration delivered to the patient. The maximum estimated oxygen concentration is 40%.

Also, to avoid drying of nasal mucosa, it is preferable to humidify the oxygen when a nasal cannula is used for hours to days or when using higher flow rates.

Infants and younger children tend to not tolerate nasal cannulas very well. For infants and younger children, oxygen cubes or oxygen hoods are available for oxygen administration. These devices are discussed next.

b. Oxygen Cube/Hood

An oxygen hood is a transparent enclosure that surrounds an infant's head. An oxygen cube surrounds both the head and the upper body. Oxygen flows (at a high flow rate of 10-15

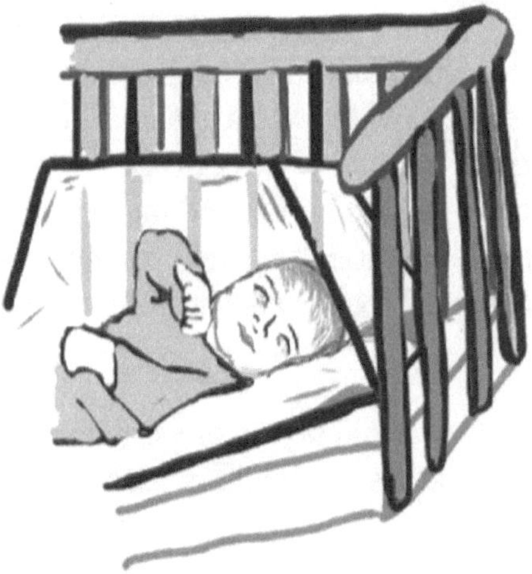

L/min) into the cube or hood via corrugated tubing that is connected to a source of oxygen. An oxygen analyzer may be used to estimate the oxygen concentration in the hood or cube. The oxygen cube/hood may be used to provide oxygen supplementation to infants and young children, but may also be used to provide high humidity to these patients. An oxygen concentration of 30 –40 % can be achieved with these devices.

c. Venti Mask

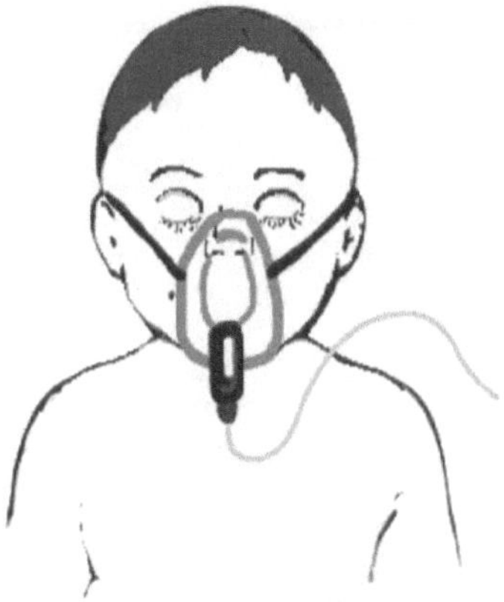

This is a full-face mask with a corrugated reservoir and specific oxygen concentration adaptor. The mask is connected to a high flow source of oxygen. By altering the flow of oxygen and the oxygen concentration adaptor the actual fraction of inspired oxygen (FiO2) may be estimated as follow:

Desired FiO2	Oxygen flow rate
0.35	8 liters/min
0.40	8 liters/min
	(The oxygen concentration adaptor is adjusted to 0.4, this will change the amount of room air entrained to keep FiO2 at 0.4)
0.5	10 liters/min

d. Partial-Rebreather Mask

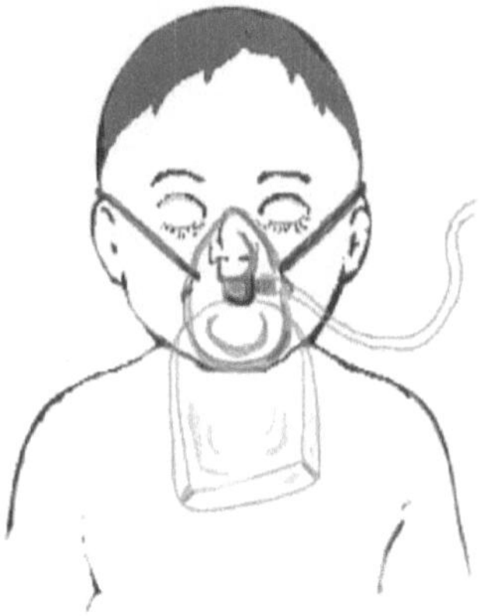

When the above oxygen devices fail to maintain satisfactory hemoglobin oxygen saturation for a patient with respiratory insufficiency, the partial rebreathing mask and the non-rebreathing mask (see below) are two additional devices that are available to provide high concentrations of oxygen,

Both of these masks consist of a full-face mask and a reservoir (a plastic bag) attached to a high flow (10-15 L/min) oxygen supply (Figure 2). A continuous source of high flow oxygen fills the reservoir at all times. Therefore it is critical to observe that the **reservoir is always inflated (full of air) when your patient is on one of these devices. The reservoir should not collapse at any point during therapy**. This device can deliver FiO2 of 0.6 – 0.8 (60 –80%).

e. Non-Rebreather Mask

The non-rebreather mask is similar to a partial-rebreather mask described above with one exception. In the partial-rebreather mask, as the patient exhales, some of the exhaled air goes into the reservoir and with each subsequent breath the patient will inhale some of that air along with the fresh air (hence the name partial-rebreather) that is coming from the oxygen source.

In the non-rebreather mask there is a one-way check valve between the mask and the reservoir so that the patient gets only fresh air from the reservoir. When the patient exhales the air is vented to the outside via a circular opening on one side of the mask. This device can deliver up to 80-100% oxygen = FiO2 0.8 - 1.0.

Sequence of oxygen therapy devices in patients with hypoxemic respiratory insufficiency:

Nasal cannula

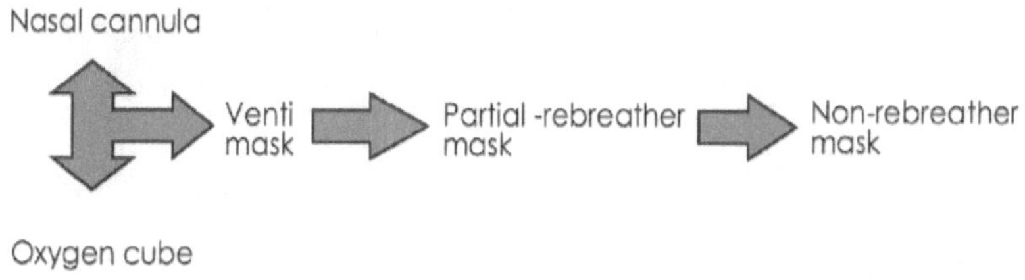

Clinical Vignette:

You have a patient on a non-rebreather mask. However, the SpO2 on pulse oximetry has a low reading of only 83%. The patient demonstrates central cyanosis. What would you do now?

You could go to a trial of non-invasive ventilation such as CPAP or BiPAP depending on your experience and the comfort level. Most of these patients will eventually need tracheal intubation and positive pressure ventilation. CPAP/BiPAP will be discussed in later sections of this pocket guide.

At this point you should have obtained an arterial blood gas to evaluate the oxygenation and ventilation status of the patient. Some of the indications for positive pressure ventilation involve analysis and interpretation of blood gases. We will discuss these indications below.

Figure 1:

Venti mask which consists of:

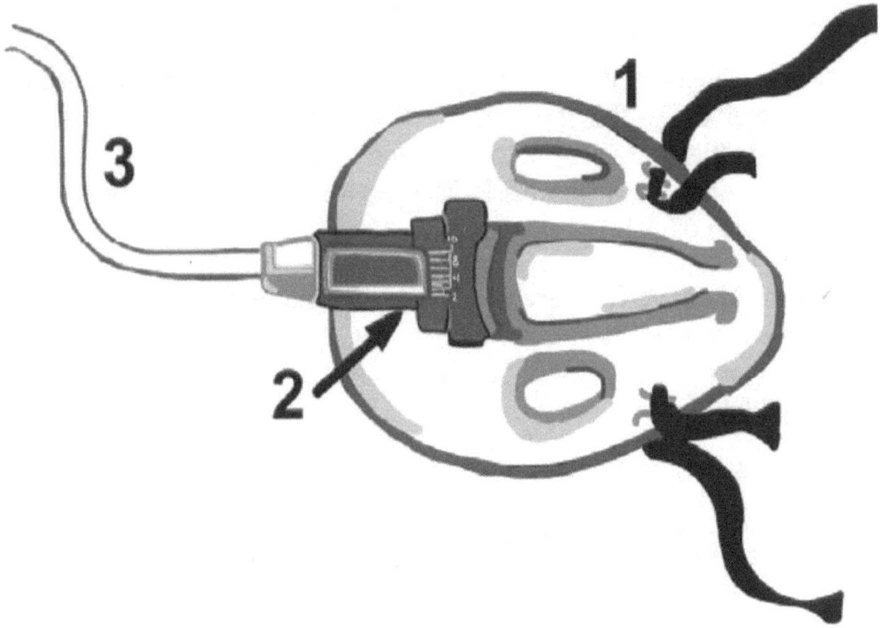

1. Face mask
2. Oxygen concentration adapter
3. The tube for the oxygen source

Figure 2:

Partial-Rebreather and Non-Rebreather mask. With a non-rebreather mask, a one-way check valve is located at point B, so that the patient inhales only fresh oxygen (80 -100% oxygen) from the oxygen reservoir.

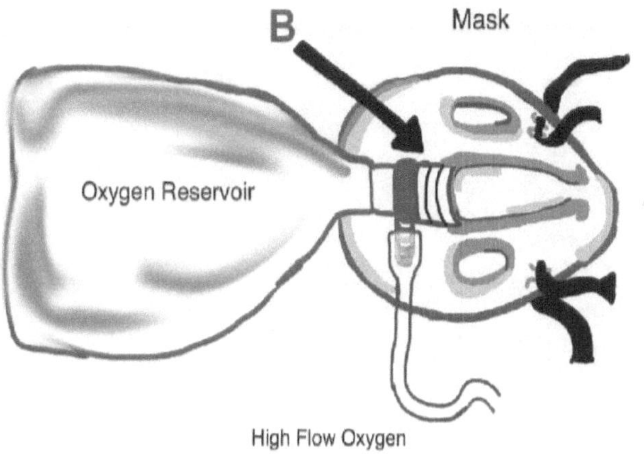
B
Mask
Oxygen Reservoir
High Flow Oxygen

Indications for Initiation of Mechanical Ventilation

In the upcoming sections of this booklet we will focus on positive pressure ventilation that is delivered to patients who are intubated (tracheal intubation via the oral route or the nasal route) or for patients who have a tracheostomy in place.

In the latter sections of this pocket guide we will also discuss non-invasive ventilation, i.e. delivery of positive pressure ventilation to patients who are not intubated such as Continuous Positive Airway Pressure (CPAP) or Bi-level Positive Airway Pressure (BiPAP).

It is important to recognize that the decision to intubate the patient and institute mechanical ventilation is a clinical one and varies from one clinical situation to another. However, in general, indications for initiation of mechanical ventilation include abnormalities in oxygenation, ventilation and others. These are discussed below:

I. Oxygenation Abnormalities

a. Inability to attain and sustain a satisfactory oxygen saturation as detected by pulse oximetry on high concentration of inspired oxygen, i.e. 80 -100%.

b. b. PaO_2 < 60 torr or central cyanosis on a high concentration of oxygen (80- 100%).

c. Alveolar-arterial oxygen gradient = P (A-a) O2 > 300 torr while the patient is receiving 100% oxygen, i.e. FiO2 1.0.

What is A-a Gradient?

The A-a gradient is the difference between the expected oxygen tension in the alveoli and the measured oxygen concentration in the arterial blood (PaO2). We calculate it as follows:

Expected alveolar Oxygen (PAO_2) = (barometric pressure – vapor pressure) X FiO_2 - $PaCO_2$ / 0.8

Let us assume that your patient is on 100% oxygen (FiO_2=1.0) and the blood gas shows:

pH	7.38
$PaCO_2$	38
PaO_2	55

Expected alveolar Oxygen
(PAO_2) = (747– 47) X 1.0 – (38/ 0.8)

= (700) – (47.5)

= 652

The arterial oxygen tension for the patient (PaO_2) is only 55 torr.

Therefore the A-a gradient is 652 – 55 = 597 torr, clearly much greater than 300.

The above indications assume that the patient is clearly in respiratory distress from a pulmonary disease.

II. Ventilation Abnormalities

a. Apnea.

b. Increased airway resistance or airway obstruction associated with hypercarbia (high $PaCO_2$; to 60s and 70s torr) leading to significant acidemia (low pH, let us say < 7.2).

c. Decreased ventilatory derive associated with a high or rapidly rising $PaCO_2$ (hypercarbia) leading to significant academia.

d. Neuromuscular diseases such as Myasthenia gravis in acute crisis, muscle dystrophies or myopathies with acute decompensation: some of these patients may be managed with CPAP/BiPAP. Remember that these patients may not be able to exhibit signs of respiratory distress because they do not have the muscle strength due to the underlying muscle weakness. In these patients we rely on two bedside pulmonary parameters to assess the need for positive pressure ventilation, namely:

   1. Forced vital capacity of < 15 ml/kg body weight.

   2. Inability to generate a negative inspiratory force of at – 20 cm H2O or more negative.

e. Edema of the chest wall as with multiple organ dysfunction and kyphoscoliosis (with a dead space to tidal volume ratio >0.6 (normal <0.3)) are both examples of respiratory muscle dysfunction and chest wall abnormalities/deformities, leading to inadequate ventilation/recruitment of pulmonary parenchyma.

f. Spinal cord injury leading the respiratory muscle weakness with ventilation abnormalities.

III. Other Indications for Positive Pressure Ventilation

Positive pressure ventilation may also be beneficial in the following clinical situations:

a. Depressed level of consciousness with the inability to protect the airway from secretions.

b. To permit sedation and paralysis in order to prevent or reduce intracranial hypertension in the setting of head injury. In this setting maintaining normoxemia and perhaps mild hyperventilation ($PaCO_2$ of 35 – 40 torr) is beneficial to the patient because these two interventions decrease cerebral blood flow, which in turn decreases intracranial pressure. However, the beneficial effects of this strategy may be short-lived (6-12 hours).

c. To decrease myocardial oxygen consumption by decreasing afterload in patients with myocardial dysfunction or congestive cardiac failure, since positive pressure reduces afterload by decreasing the transmural pressure across the aorta.

d. To decrease systemic oxygen consumption in patients with multiple organ dysfunction syndrome.

e. To institute Positive End-Expiratory Pressure (PEEP) in order to prevent dependent lung atelectasis.

Positive Pressure Ventilation (PPV)

The purpose of Positive Pressure Ventilation is to provide the force necessary for the generation of tidal breath and to alter and optimize the end-expiratory lung volume in order to improve oxygenation. The lung volume at the end of normal spontaneous exhalation is called the functional residual capacity (FRC), as shown in **Figure 3**. In this figure: the Y-axis is flow in liters and the X-axis is time in seconds.

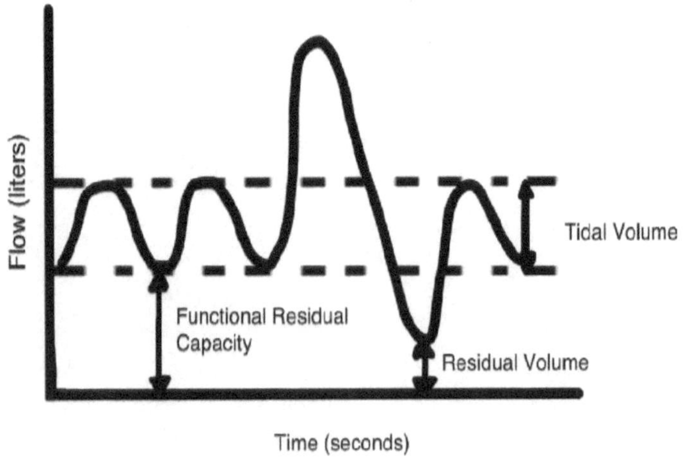

Figure 3

Functional Residual Capacity (FRC) is the lung volume that is critical for oxygenation. With most pulmonary alveolar diseases (such as pneumonia, ARDS) that lead to hypoxemia the FRC is reduced. In order to improve oxygenation after positive pressure ventilation is initiated one needs to employ strategies that will increase and optimize the FRC. This may be accomplished by either increasing and optimizing Mean Airway Pressure (MAP) or the Transpulmonary Pressure (TPP). The TPP = alveolar pressure – pleural pressure. The TPP is difficult to measure in the day-to-day practice in the intensive care unit. Therefore, we will focus on the MAP. As we will discuss next, a major component of the MAP is Positive End-Expiratory Pressure (PEEP). PEEP is the constant pressure that is applied during the exhalation phase of the respiratory cycle in order to open the alveoli and maintain their patency throughout the respiratory cycle. This is called recruitment and is a major mechanism that improves FRC and this in turn improves oxygenation.

Figure 4

Overview of the theoretically proposed outcome of PEEP application during Positive Pressure Ventilation.

Inspiration begins at **POINT A** with the application of positive pressure and this pressure reaches a peak called the **Peak Inspiratory Pressure (PIP).** The pressure is sustained for the duration of inspiration and this time period is appropriately named the **Inspiratory Time (IT)**.

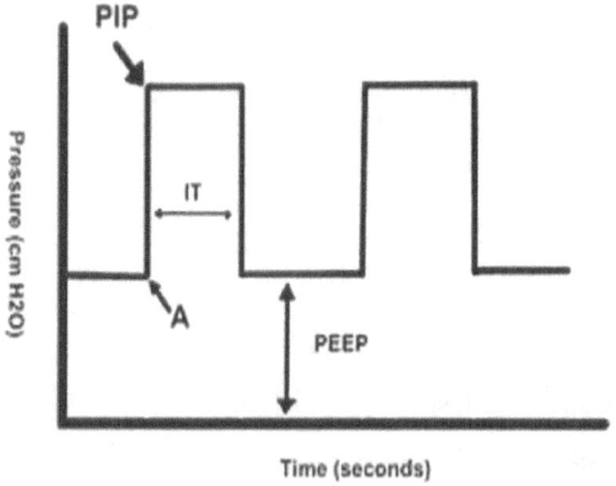

Figure 4: Overview of the theoretically proposed outcome of PEEP application during Positive Pressure Ventilation.

In reality the pressure dissipates early during inspiration and drops to a lower pressure level called the plateau pressure (discussed later).

Then the pressure drops back to where it started as exhalation begins. This pressure sustained throughout the exhalation phase is called the

Positive End-Expiratory Pressure (PEEP). Note: as you can see it is a misnomer, but has been called PEEP for decades and we continue to call it PEEP.

The plateau pressure is more difficult to measure and is not as readily available on most ventilator screens and so we will use the PIP for the calculation of the MAP.

The approximate MAP is the area under the curve in **Figure 4**. The area under curve = the area of the individual (if you can imagine them in figure 4) rectangles (which represent individual breaths) plus the area under the long horizontal rectangle (which represents PEEP).

The area of individual vertical rectangles = height of each rectangle

= (PIP – PEEP) X IT

= length of each rectangle.

Therefore:

$$MAP = \frac{(PIP - PEEP) \times IT \times RR}{60} + PEEP$$

We explain this equation as follows:

1. (PIP – PEEP) X IT : This represents the area of individual vertical rectangles. The pressure is expressed in cm H_2O and the inspiratory time is expressed in seconds.

2. RR (respiratory or ventilatory rate) is expressed in breaths per minute = total number of vertical rectangles per minute

3. 60: is a mathematical factor since the IT is in seconds and the RR is in number of breaths per minute. There are 60 seconds in a minute, hence the factor of 60.

4. PEEP is the pressure that always is there throughout the respiratory cycle.

Let us use an example from a patient on Positive Pressure Ventilation to calculate the MAP.

This patient is receiving Positive Pressure Ventilation with PIP of 30 cm H_2O, PEEP 10 cm H_2O, IT 0.5 seconds and a ventilatory rate of 20 bpm.

$$MAP = \frac{(30\text{-}10)\ X\ 0.5\ X\ 20}{60} + 10 = 13.3\ cm\ H_2O$$

With most current ventilators the MAP is readily available and is usually displayed on the ventilator monitor screen. However, recognizing how the MAP is derived and calculated is very helpful in understanding why we manipulate the different parameters on the ventilator for hypoxemic respiratory failure in order to improve oxygenation. All the interventions are aimed at optimizing the MAP because there is good correlation between the MAP and oxygenation. As you can see from the MAP equation, increasing PEEP is the most effective way to increase MAP since PEEP is the only parameter in the MAP equation that is a whole number. An increase in PEEP leads to a proportionate increase in MAP and they have an almost one to one relationship.

Inspiratory Time (IT)

Each breath, either spontaneous or ventilator assisted, consists of inspiration and exhalation (expiration) with a normal ratio of inspiration (IT) to expiration (expiratory time). The normal ratio for inspiration to expiration (I:E) is approximately 1:2 for children and 1:3 for adults. As we will discuss in later sections, Positive Pressure Ventilation may be accomplished using volume or pressure as the primary parameters. When we use pressure we also set the IT. For example we could set an IT of 0.7 seconds. If the ventilatory rate is set at 20 bpm, this means that the total respiratory cycle (inspiration and expiration = 3 seconds); of this 0.7 is for inspiration and 3 – 0.7 = 2.3 seconds for expiration. Therefore the I:E would be approximately 1:3.

With volume ventilation we usually do not set the inspiratory time. In this type of ventilation the IT is a function of the flow through the ventilatory circuit. This is something we have not discussed yet and you may find it confusing, but be patient you will understand all these issues as you progress through this booklet.

When a ventilator delivers positive pressure breaths to a patient there is a more or less constant flow of air/oxygen through the ventilatory circuit that varies depending on the patient's age and size. This is called flow. A respiratory therapist usually sets this flow based on age and size of the patient. That is why if you are a physician, you are usually not asked to set this variable as a parameter, but it is an important parameter to understand and we will discuss it further in a later section. Let us get back to the IT with volume ventilation. In this setting the IT is a function of the flow. Let us say that you are ventilating a patient with a tidal volume of 500 mL and the flow through the ventilator circuit is set and 50 liters/min. The IT will be as follows:

50 liters = 50,000 mL delivered in 60 seconds Therefore, 500 mL will be delivered in 0.6 seconds. The IT in this patient will be 0.6 seconds with each ventilator – delivered breath.

Let us get back the Mean Airway Pressure (MAP) for a moment. Remember, we discussed that PEEP was the major component of the MAP that increases the MAP most effectively (they have almost a one to one relationship). The next parameter that is used to increase MAP is the IT. As you increase the IT the MAP increases, but the I:E also changes. Let us take the example above where the IT was set at 0.7 and ventilatory rate was 20 bpm.

The initial I:E	will be 1:2	at 20 bpm, and an IT = 0.7
The subsequent I:E	will be 1:1	at 20 bpm, if IT = 1.5 sec
**** The I:E**	**will be 2:1**	**at 20 bpm, if IT= 2.0 sec**

So, for a patient on Positive Pressure Ventilation for hypoxemic respiratory failure, in order to improve oxygenation, you need to take the following steps:

1. Increase the oxygen concentration (FiO_2) within a safe range i.e. < 0.6 or 60% oxygen (see table here).

2. Increase the MAP gradually by increasing PEEP by 1 - 2 increments according to the guidelines in the table here. Then you can gradually increase the IT.

3. You may increase the IT by 0.1 – 0.2 seconds until you reach an acceptable I:E ratio. You may increase the IT until you reach inverse ration ventilation and we will discuss this further at a later section.

4. Oxygenation generally improves as the MAP is increased until approximately 25 cm H_2O. Generally there is minimal further improvement in oxygenation when MAP is increased beyond this level. We will discuss this further in the section below.

There are other factors that affect manipulation of the ventilatory parameters in order to improve MAP and hence oxygenation. Table 1 below shows a summary of the guidelines for optimizing MAP in patients with acute hypoxemic respiratory failure.

The required MAP will depend on the extent of lung injury (determined by PaO2/FiO2) and patient's chest wall compliance (decreased in patients with obesity, edema as a result of extensive fluid resuscitation, and abdominal distension). The parameter that is most effective in increasing MAP is PEEP. Gradually increase FiO2 and PEEP according to **Table 1** below to achieve an oxygen saturation of 88-93%.

Table 1: Shows one suggested guideline for improving oxygenation in patients with hypoxemic respiratory failure.

FiO2 required to maintain target SpO2	Chest wall compliance	
	Normal	Decreased
0.3	PEEP = 5	10
0.4	8	12
0.5	10	14
0.6	12	16

Higher levels of PEEP has been recommended in older children and adults when higher FiO2 is required to maintain a satisfactory oxygen saturation. However, one has to be careful with higher levels of PEEP because of associated hemodynamic problems. At these higher levels of PEEP consider other measures to increase the MAP, such as increasing the IT, or the PIP (or tidal volume). In general PIP and tidal are not commonly used to improve MAP since increasing the PIP or tidal volume is more likely to be associated with barotrauma.

Volume or Pressure?

When using Positive Pressure Ventilation for a patient with respiratory insufficiency we choose one of two general approaches of volume or pressure. In volume ventilation the tidal volume (TV) is preset while in the pressure ventilation the peak inspiratory pressure (PIP) is preset. Most of the other parameters are the same with both approaches with few exceptions. When Positive Pressure Ventilation is initiated in a patient you will have to prescribe a number of parameters that will determine oxygenation and ventilation. These parameters are as follows depending on whether you are using volume or pressure ventilation:

	Volume Ventilation	Pressure Ventilation
Oxygenation	FiO_2	FiO_2
	PEEP	PEEP
	Inspiratory Time (IT)	Inspiratory Time (IT)
Ventilation	Tidal Volume	PIP
	Ventilatory Rate	Ventilatory Rate

Table 2

By now you should know the elements that determine the MAP, namely PEEP, IT, PIP, and ventilatory rate. Also you will know by now that PEEP and IT are the main parameters that are most effective in optimizing the MAP. Furthermore, the IT is a parameter that is set by the practitioner in the pressure type of ventilation, while where the IT is a function of the flow, volume type of ventilation is usually not set by the practitioner.

Volume Ventilation

Tidal volume: is the volume of air/oxygen that is delivered to the patient with each breath. The volume is selected as mL/kg body weight. Based on research results over the past 10-15 years, which has shown that lung injury correlates with high tidal volume (10-15 mL/kg), the current recommendation is to use low tidal volume ventilation (5-8 mL/kg). After you have selected a tidal volume for your patient, how do you evaluate whether the tidal volume is adequate both clinically and on blood gases?

Clinically one looks for adequacy of chest expansion and the presence of satisfactory breath sounds both centrally and peripherally. On blood gases one looks for an acceptable pH and $PaCO_2$.

Advantages of Low Tidal Volume Ventilation

It appears that low tidal volume ventilation when combined with high PEEP produces excellent gas exchange by bringing the FRC and the compliance of the respiratory system close towards normal while reducing the so called cyclic stretching of the lungs which is believed to be responsible for lung injury. **What is cyclic stretching anyway?**

In patients with hypoxemic respiratory failure such as ARDS the alveoli in the diseased areas of the lungs are collapsed and are opened with each inspiration when a preset tidal volume is delivered to the lungs. When inspiration ends and expiration begins these alveoli return to a collapsed state, but are "ripped" open with the next cycle of inspiration. Each time these lung units are ripped open with a mechanical breath there is a possibility of damage to the lung units followed by lung inflammation. One way to keep the diseased lung units open is to apply a constant pressure that is high enough to keep these units open throughout the respiratory cycle, and to superimpose on this, small tidal breaths that will with ventilation. This is precisely what is done in the strategy of high PEEP, low tidal volume ventilation. When high PEEP (see Table 1 for guidelines on use of PEEP) is used, the diseased and collapsed alveolar units are opened and kept open throughout the respiratory cycle (as opposed to collapsing during expiration, which may occur with use of lower PEEP) and are ventilated with small tidal volume.

Pressure Ventilation

In pressure ventilation the Peak Inspiratory Pressure (PIP) is the parameter that replaces the tidal volume. One may select a PIP that produces a tidal volume of 5-8 mL/kg body weight in order to avoid high tidal volume ventilation. Most current ventilators display (on a screen) the tidal volume that corresponds to the PIP that is being delivered to the patient. By the same token, these ventilators will also display the PIP that corresponds to the tidal volume that is being delivered to the patient when the patient is receiving volume ventilation. So if you are not certain where to start the PIP with your patient, one option you have is to deliver a tidal volume of 5-8 mL/kg for a brief period and observe the corresponding PIP that is needed to deliver the particular tidal volume. Then switch the patient to pressure ventilation with the appropriate PIP. Again, the adequacy of the PIP is determined by the adequacy of chest expansion and good air entry both centrally and peripherally. Again if you are not sure where to start with PIP when you initiate pressure ventilation, you may use the following guidelines:

Neonates ⟶ start with PIP of 20 cm H_2O
Infants ⟶ start with PIP of low to mid 20s
Toddlers ⟶ start with PIP in the mid 20s
Older child ⟶ start with PIP high 20s
Adolescents/ ⟶ start with PIP in the
adults ⟶ low 30s

Subsequently you may adjust the PIP by 1-2 cm H_2O up or down to achieve the appropriate tidal volume based on chest expansion, air entry, and results of blood gases.

Pressure ventilation is also referred to as pressure control ventilation and time-cycled pressure-limited ventilation depending on the type of ventilator one is using. In pressure control ventilation, the pressure control refers to the difference between the PIP and PEEP. So, if the PIP is 30 and PEEP is 10, then the pressure control of 20 cm H_2O.

As we stated earlier with pressure ventilation, the practitioner will set the inspiratory time (IT). Start with a low IT such 0.4 or 0.5 and depending on the ventilatory rate you are using, try to maintain an I:E ratio that is closest to that of the patient being ventilated. We will discuss this in the sections below.

Thus the main parameters that are different between the volume and pressure ventilation are: Tidal Volume (TV) vs. PIP, and inspiratory time. The other parameters: FiO_2 , PEEP, and the ventilator rate are the same in both approaches. In general, pressure ventilation is used more commonly in children and volume ventilation is used more frequently in adults. Pressure ventilation in the form of time-cycled pressure limited ventilation is commonly used in neonates and infants less than 10 kg body weight.

Clinical Vignette:

Let us use an example of a 4-year-old child who is intubated for respiratory insufficiency and who needs Positive Pressure Ventilation. What settings would you prescribe if you choose to use volume ventilation? how about if you decide to use pressure ventilation for the same patient, what initial settings would you prescribe?

	Volume Ventilation	Pressure Ventilation
Oxygenation	FiO_2 = 1.0*	FiO_2 = 1.0*
	PEEP = 5cm H_2O	PEEP = 5cm H_2O
	N/A	IT = 0.5 sec
Ventilation	TV = 120 mL	PIP = 25cm H_2O
	Ventilatory Rate = 20 bpm	Ventilatory Rate = 20 bpm

Table 3

Where to Start with the Ventilatory Settings when you initiate PPV in Pediatric Patients:

A. **Neonates/Infants:**

1. Oxygen: 21 – 100%: depending on the clinical situation. Patients who are intubated for disorders other than hypoxemic respiratory failure such as depressed mental status usually require low levels of oxygen closer to 21% = room air. If you

start with high concentration of oxygen, wean the oxygen as rapidly as possible to < 60% = $FiO_2 < 0.6$ or the lowest level that will maintain a satisfactory oxygen saturation on the pulse oximetry (generally 88 – 93%).

2. PIP of 20 or a tidal volume of 5 - 8 ml/kg body weight, then adjust the PIP by 1 to 2 or the tidal volume by 1 mL/kg to maintain good chest expansion, good air entry and an acceptable $PaCO_2$ and pH.

3. PEEP of 4 -5 cm H_2O.

Ventilatory rate: 40 bpm. Adjust the rate based on the arterial $PaCO_2$.

Remember that $PaCO_2$ is affected by TV or PIP and the ventilatory rate. Once you have established that the TV or PIP are appropriately based on chest expansion and air entry. Subsequent fine tuning of the $PaCO_2$ is accomplished by manipulating the ventilatory rate according the following formula:

$$\text{Current rate X Current } PaCO_2 = \text{Desired } PaCO_2 \text{ X expected rate}$$

For example if the patient has $PaCO_2$ of 50 mm Hg on a ventilatory rate of 20 bpm and you desire to lower the $PaCO_2$ to 40 mm Hg, then the expected ventilatory rate would be:

$$50 \text{ mm Hg X } 20 \text{ bpm} = 40 \text{ mm Hg X expected rate}$$

$$\text{Expected rate} = \frac{50 \text{ mm Hg X } 20 \text{ bpm}}{40 \text{ mm Hg}} = 25 \text{ bpm}$$

This equation may be used in patients of all age groups including adults to calculate the expected ventilatory rate when attempting to adjust the $PaCO_2$.

B. **Toddlers/younger children:**

1. Oxygen: 21-100%

2. PIP: mid 20s ; adjust by 1- 2 to desired effect
3. Tidal volume (TV): 5 – 8 mL/kg body weight
4. PEEP: start at 5 cm H_2O and increase by 1-2 to desired effect
5. Ventilatory rate: 20 – 30 bpm and adjust by 5 up or down to desired effect

C. Older children up to adolescent years:

1. FiO_2 : 0.21 – 1.0
2. PIP: high 20s
3. TV 5-8 mL/kg body weight
4. PEEP: start at 5 cm H_2O and increase by 1-2 to desired effect
5. Ventilatory rate: high teens to low twenties

D. Adolescents:

1. FiO_2 : 0.21 – 1.0
2. PIP: high 20s – low 30s.
3. TV 5-8 mL/kg ideal body weight
4. PEEP: start at 5 cm H_2O and increase by 1-2 to desired effect.
5. Ventilatory rate: low to mid teens.

To adjust the ventilatory rate, please refer to the equation above. To optimize oxygenation, the following strategy is an option:

1. Increase PEEP in increments of 1 – 2 cm H_2O (in order to increase mean airway pressure [MAP]). You should know by now that when you increase PEEP by 1, MAP will also increase by 1 (see Mean

Airway Pressure equation). You may also increase FiO_2 in the safe range (< 0.6). At times it may become necessary to increase FiO_2 beyond this range. **Please see Table 1.**

2. PEEP tends to be more effective as it is increased from mid to high single digits. As PEEP reaches low teens its effect on improving oxygenation becomes somewhat more flat (Figure 5).

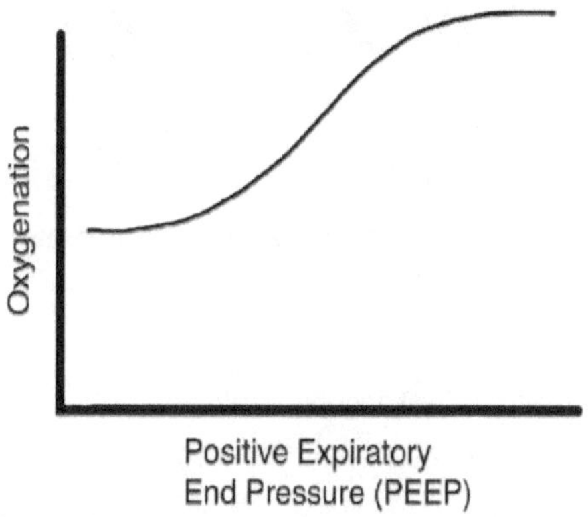

Figure 5: Effects of PEEP on oxygenation

Higher levels of PEEP may sometimes be effective in maintaining the alveoli in diseased lung units inflated, and thus avoid the cyclic stretching that was discussed earlier. This may also improve the compliance of the respiratory system and move the compliance curve (which is the relationship between pressure and volume) to a more favorable position in **Figure 6**.

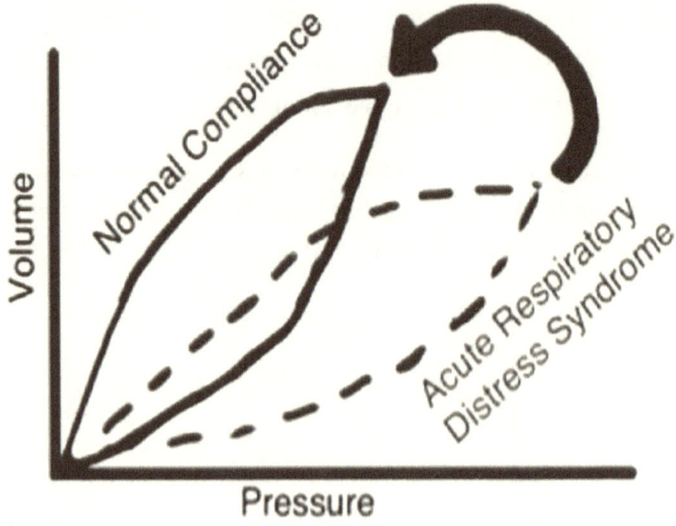

Figure 6: The relationship between pressure and volume (compliance). Increasing PEEP (up to a certain level) may move the curve to a more favorable position.

Progressively increasing PEEP may have a deleterious effect on the hemodynamic status of the patient! What does that mean? As intrathoracic pressure increases with higher PEEP, venous return may decrease, which may lead to a decrease in cardiac output. This is particularly likely if the intravascular volume status is inadequate. More recent work on this subject suggest that the cardiac output does not decrease as much as originally thought if the patient is optimally volume repleted before increasing PEEP to higher levels.

So far we have discussed PEEP and the MAP as the two determinants of oxygenation. There is another pressure called the Transpulmonary Pressure (TPP) which is the difference between the alveolar pressure and the pleural pressure:

$$\text{TPP} = \text{alveolar pressure} - \text{pleural pressure}$$

As you can see both these pressures are difficult to measure at the bedside for the day-to-day clinical practice of medicine. The esophageal pressure can approximate the pleural pressure. In this method a balloon-tipped catheter is inserted in the lower part of the esophagus and the pressure that is measured will approximate the pleural pressure. The alveolar pressure is of course difficult, if not impossible, to measure (but can be measured in experimental methods of lung mechanics).

In experimental models of the lung, it has been shown that the lungs are maximally distended at a TPP of 35 cm H_2O. If you exceed this pressure limit (when the lungs are maximally distended) all you will be doing is causing over distention of the lungs, particularly the healthy units. Possibly resulting in barotraumas and further lung injury.

In practice, another pressure that can be measured on most ventilators is the plateau pressure. As we discussed earlier, during inspiration the pressure increases to reach the time at 0.6 second, the ventilator will switch from inspiration to expiration after 0.6 seconds.

The plateau pressure is the pressure that occupies most of the inspiration. This pressure may be obtained on most current ventilators by dialing in a long inspiratory pause (usually done by the respiratory therapist who should be able to provide you this pressure if you ask for it). Because measurements of the alveolar pressure and pleural pressure are not possible at the bedside in the day-to-day practice of medicine, the plateau pressure has been used as an approximate pressure for the TPP.

The plateau pressure is a useful pressure that has been used in clinical practice to avoid overdistention and lung injuries. It is recommended that (in the mature lung) the plateau pressure be limited to 35 cm H_2O. In clinical situations where chest wall stiffness is suspected, and the lung is mature, it is acceptable to increase the plateau pressure upper limit to 40 cm H_2O.

If you notice beaking at the upper portion of the compliance curve, this suggests ongoing over distention of the lungs (Figure 7). This means there is no further recruitment or volume generated once we exceed a certain pressure limit. This lack of recruitment or volume expansion with application of additional pressure is referred to as overdistention. The pressure-volume curve is readily available on most current ventilators and may be observed continuously on the ventilator monitor.

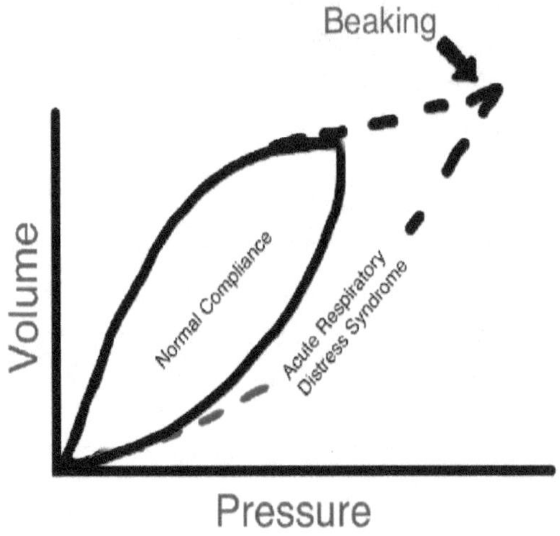

Figure 7 Pressure-Volume curve showing pulmonary compliance. With over distention, beaking is noted at high pressures, suggesting that there is no further increase in volume as the pressure in increased.

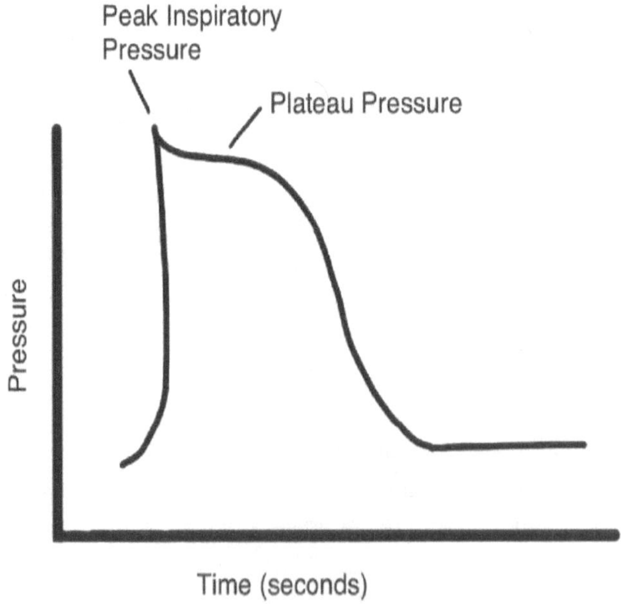

Figure 8: Shows the peak inspiratory pressure (PIP) and the plateu pressure on a pressure-time curve from a conventional ventilator.

Positive Pressure Ventilation (PPV) in Adults

Most ventilatory support in adult patients is accomplished with volume-cycled ventilation, as opposed to pressure ventilation in children. The cycling designation refers to the parameter that determines the end of inspiratory phase. With pressure ventilation it is the inspiratory time (set by the practitioner) that terminates inspiration. If you set the inspiratory time at 0.6 second, the ventilator will switch from inspiration to expiration after 0.6 seconds.

With volume cycled ventilation what is the parameter that determines cycling between the inspiration and expiration?

The answer is the tidal volume. When a preset tidal volume e.g. 500 mL is reached, inspiration ends and exhalation begins and the ventilator will switch from inspiration to expiration.

What determines the Inspiratory Time (IT) in volume cycled ventilation?

As we discussed earlier, with volume ventilation the flow of air/oxygen that circulates through the ventilatory circuit determines the IT. The flow rate is generally set at 60 – 90 liters/min for adult patients, depending on the underlying clinical condition. In general, patients with pulmonary alveolar diseases such as ARDS need lower flow rates, while patients with airway disease such as asthma or Chronic Obstructive Pulmonary Disease (COPD) need higher flow rates.

Higher flow rates translates into a longer total ventilatory cycle and the tidal volume will be delivered to the patient faster, (i.e. shorter IT) which in turn translates into a longer expiratory time. Patients with airway disease (obstruction), such as asthma and COPD, need a longer exhalation time and hence they need a higher flow (closer to 90 liters/minute). Let us use an example to illustrate this concept:

Clinical Vignette

A 65-year-old male is intubated for respiratory failure due to COPD exacerbation. he is receiving a tidal volume of 800 mL and a ventilatory rate of 15 bpm. The flow through the ventilatory circuit is set at 48 liters/min. What is the IT and the I:E ratio?

48 liters = 48,000 ml is delivered over one minute = 60 seconds

Therefore, 800 ml will delivered over X seconds = IT

X = IT = 500 X 60 / 60,000 = 1.0 second.

The patient is receiving 15 bpm

Therefore, the total ventilatory cycle = 4 seconds (60/15 = 4)

IT = 1. 0 and the ET would be 3.0; with an I:E of 1:3.

With this ratio there may not be sufficient time for exhalation considering the patient has airway obstructive disease. The airways are inflamed and narrowed with an increased resistance to airflow, which will lead to delayed emptying of the lungs.

If we increase the flow rate from 48 to 90 liters/min, what IT and I:E will we get?

IT = 0.53 second

Since the rate is the same, the total ventilatory time is still 4 seconds and so the time left for exhalation would be 4 – 0.5 =3.5 seconds and the I:E 1:7. So now the patient has longer time for exhalation.

In patients with obstructive lung diseases, such as asthma and COPD, a flow-time curve is one way to graphically monitor adequacy of exhalation time, which are available on most ventilators.

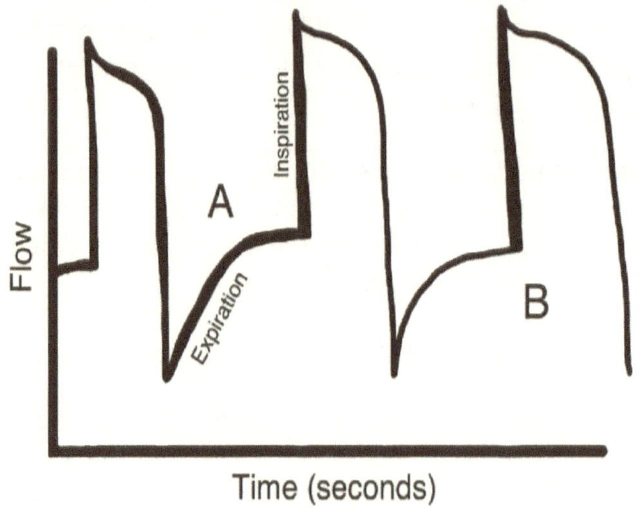

Figure 9

During breath **A**, the flow of the **expiratory phase** does reach the baseline, before the next breath. In this case there is adequate time for exhalation. Meaning the lungs were able to deflate and reach baseline volume before the next breath initiated. However, in breath **B**, exhalation flow does not reach the baseline (diamond) before the next breath. Depicting there was not adequate time for exhalation. Recurrence of this problem can lead to "stacking of breaths" and the phenomenon of air trapping, which may result in pneumothorax and/or pneumomediastinum.

As discussed earlier, with volume ventilation the current recommendation is to use a tidal volume of 5 – 8 ml/kg body weight. When using volume ventilation this tidal volume has a corresponding pressure (that is necessary to deliver this tidal volume). The level of this pressure will vary depending on the underlying condition of the patient. If one is ventilating a normal or healthy lung, the pressure that is necessary to deliver a tidal volume of 5 – 8 ml/kg is usually not significant -- perhaps in the high teens to low twenties. However, if we attempt to ventilate a disease lung, (parenchymal disease such ARDS or airway disease such as asthma) the pressure (PIP or the plateau pressure) that may be necessary to deliver a tidal volume may be significantly higher and sometimes may reach unacceptable levels such as a PIP of > 50 cm H_2O or a plateau pressure of > 35 cm H_2O. These high pressures can potentially lead to complications such pneumomediastinum and/or pneumothorax. If you see the above flow-time pattern in your patient, you need to change the ventilator settings so that you allow the patient to have a longer exhalation time: by increasing the flow rate or decreasing the ventilatory rate or both.

How do I avoid high airway pressures in my patients who are on volume-cycled ventilation?

High inspiratory airway pressure (PIP > 50 cm H_2O or a plateau pressure > 35 cm H_2O) are of concern because of the risks of pulmonary barotraumas and air leakage such as pneumomediastinum and/or pneumothorax. Strategies that may be used to minimize these complications include:

1. Decrease the flow through the ventilatory circuit:

from laws of physics: **pressure = flow X resistance**

Therefore, if flow is decreased, the pressure should also decrease. However, this may be a problem in patients with obstructive lung disease because of the associated reduction in expiratory time. Like we discussed earlier, flow is not a parameter that will likely be asked of you if you're a physician, because the respiratory therapist usually sets the flow rate. However, it is an important concept to understand.

There are few patterns for the flow through the ventilatory circuit. The most important of which is the **decelerating flow,** which means there is a very high flow rate at the beginning of inspiration until the flow reaches a peak flow (of let us say 60 liters per minute), then the flow decelerates. This decelerating flow pattern is the most commonly used type of flow and it is believed to be associated with a more uniform distribution of ventilation in patients with lungs diseases that require Positive Pressure Ventilation. This decelerating flow pattern is shown in Figure 8.

2. Decrease the Tidal Volume (TV): to a lower level or to as low as possible. This may produce hypercarbia because of the associated reduction in minute ventilation. Minute ventilation = Tidal Volume X ventilatory rate, and so a decrease in Tidal Volume will lead to a decrease in minute ventilation. Most practitioners currently accept higher levels of carbon dioxide in exchange for lower peak pressures since the latter is associated with barotruama and lung injury and it has also been shown to improve outcome in patients with hypoxemic respiratory failure. This concept is called permissive hypercarbia and refers to the process of allowing the carbon dioxide to increase above and beyond what has been considered normal ranges for $PaCO_2$ (35 – 45 mm Hg).

How far you should allow the carbon dioxide to increase in the blood is a matter of experience, comfort level, and the clinical situations, but $PaCO_2$ in the high 50s and a pH in the 7.2 range are commonly practiced in the critical care arena provided there are no contraindications to elevation of carbon dioxide such increased intracranical pressure.

Clinical Guidelines for PPV in Adults to Limit Regional Lung Unit Over Distention:

Initially:

A tidal volume of 5 - 8 ml/kg with a decelerating inspiratory flow (60 –80 liters/min) pattern.

Timing	Oxygenation	Chest Radiograph	Pulmonary Artery Occlusion Pressure
Acute onset	PaO2/ FiO2 < 300 Regardless of PEEP level*	Bilateral infiltratres with a normal heart size	< 18 mm Hg or no evidence of left atrial hypertension level

* Start with a PEEP of 5 and increase by 1 - 2 to maintain a $PaO_2 > 60$ torr on

FiO_2 £ 0.6 and adjust the PEEP upward to an MAP of 25 cm H_2O.

Start with a ventilatory rate of 10 – 12 bpm. Adjust the ventilatory rate to avoid primary acid-base imbalances.

Subsequently:

If hypoxemia persists (PaO_2 < 60 torr): go to a trial of MAP > 25 cm H_2O or decrease the plateau pressure to < 35 cm H_2O by decreasing the inspiratory flow rate, tidal volume, or PEEP in that order.

In cases of unilateral pulmonary alveolar disease, single lung ventilation should also be considered.

Detailed discussion of single lung ventilation is beyond the scope of this pocket guide.

Ventilatory Guidelines for Specific Clinical Situations in Adult Patients:

1. ***Acute Respiratory Distress Syndrome (ARDS):*** is a complex parenchymal lung disease with severe hypoxemia with multiple causes and clinical courses. The American-European Consensus Criteria for ARDS are as follows:

*Some call PaO_2/FiO_2 < 300, acute lung injury and a PaO_2/FiO_2 < 200 ARDS.

The major goals of PPV in these patients are to maintain adequate oxygenation while avoiding high inspiratory airway pressure, high oxygen concentration, and decreasing work of breathing. Work of breathing is increased in ARDS due to markedly decreased compliance of the lungs.

For ARDS a lung protective strategy called **open lung strategy** has been suggested to minimize lung injury from PPV. This principle of the open lung strategy is similar to all the principles that we have discussed so far in this pocket guide. Namely recruiting alveoli by applying adequate (but not excessive) pressure, and avoiding high plateau pressure in order to avoid cyclic stretching and to maintain adequate oxygenation at an acceptable fraction of inspired oxygen.

This **open lung strategy** may be implemented on one brand of ventilators called **Servo *i*Ò**

as follows:

1. Use the pressure control mode on the ventilator and record baseline values for tidal volume, compliance, heart rate, blood pressure and monitor these parameters closely.

2. Increase the PEEP in increments of 3 - 5 to 18 - 20 cm H_2O.

3. Increase the peak pressure or delta P (PIP – PEEP) in 5 cm H_2O increments while closely monitoring the blood pressure (looking for hypotension) and the compliance. Continue to increase the pressure (up to 40 – 50 cm H_2O) until the compliance decreases. This means that you have reached a point of over distension = the baked portion of the compliance shown in Figure 7. Maintain these settings for approximately two minutes (if the blood pressure is stable) and then gradually decrease the peak pressure.

4. Decrease the delta P until the desired tidal volume (5 – 8 ml/kg ideal body weight) is reached. You may notice an increase in the compliance which indicates that overdistension is being relieved.

5. Slowly decrease PEEP while monitoring the compliance. You may notice that compliance increases, indicating relief of overdistention. As you decrease the PEEP further you may notice a drop in compliance indicating the beginning of lung collapse. Identify (using a cursor on the ventilator monitor such the Servo *i*ä) the optimum PEEP that produces the best compliance. Maintain the PEEP at 2 - 4 cm H_2O above the PEEP that produces the best compliance.

2. *Obstructive lung diseases including chronic Obstructive Pulmonary Disease (COPD) and asthma.* Mechanical ventilation in patients with COPD and asthma is directed at supporting oxygenation and assisting with ventilation until the airway obstruction improves.

Positive Pressure Ventilation in these patients often produces hyperinflation (with auto-PEEP) and air trapping and it may be associated with hypotension after intubation and initiation of mechanical ventilation.

Hypotension following intubation is a serious clinical problem and can be fatal if not recognized and treated promptly. It can be treated effectively and immediately by the administration of intravenous fluid to expand intravascular volume, as well as decreasing the tidal volume or the peak inspiratory pressures.

The initial tidal volume should be in the range of 5 - 8 ml/kg, and the minute ventilation should be adjusted to an acceptable pH level. Attention, however, should be given to the flow rates and the inspiratory to expiratory ratio in order to maximize the expiratory time and allow complete exhalation before the next inspiratory cycle begins. This would require higher levels of flow through the ventilatory circuit.

Flow is a parameter that you as a practitioner (or a trainee) infrequently will be asked about. But it refers to the flow of gas through the ventilatory circuit and is expressed in liters per minute (L/min). For adult patients it ranges from 50 – 90 L/min. At this time it is helpful to discuss (again) the flow as an important parameter during Positive Pressure Ventilation. Usually the respiratory therapist sets the flow rate based on the patients' underlying lung condition. In order to better understand the flow, it is helpful to understand the concept of time constant. Time constant (Tc) is the amount of time it takes the air to move from one place to another within the tracheobronchial tree. Patients with increased airway resistance have a longer time constant because it takes them longer to move air throughout the tracheobronchial tree. Therefore, they need a higher flow rate. A higher flow rate means the tidal volume will be delivered to the lungs faster, which translates into a faster inspiratory time and therefore there will be more time for exhalation. Patients with obstructive lungs diseases such COPD and asthma need longer exhalation time and hence they need higher flow rates. Generally the flow rate needs to be closer to 90 L/min as opposed to 60 L/min. However, from basic laws of physics we know that:

$$\text{Pressure} = \text{flow X resistance}$$

Therefore, if flow is increased (and assuming the resistance remains constant), the pressure is likely to increase. Therefore, in patients with COPD and asthma, if the flow is increased significantly, the peak inspiratory pressure may increase.

If the flow rates are too high, leading to an increase in inspiratory pressure (of let's say greater than 50 cm H_2O) that *can* potentially increase the risk of barotrauma and lung injury. If you are faced with this situation, the alternative is to decrease the tidal volume or ventilatory rate in order to increase the expiratory time. In fact one of the most effective ways of increasing the expiratory time in these patients is to decrease the ventilation rate to 10 or even 8 breaths per minute. Decreasing the rate is more effective in increasing the expiratory time compared to decreasing the flow.

Here is how changing the flow rate or the ventilatory rate can increase exhalation time and allow more time for exhalation. Let us take an example of a 70-kg patient who is receiving a tidal volume of 500 ml and a flow rate of 50 L/min at a rate of 20 breaths per minute.

50,000 ml in 1 min = 60 seconds

500 ml will be delivered in X seconds

X = 500 X 60 / 50,000 = 0.6 seconds

In other words the inspiratory time in this patient will be 0.6 seconds. At the ventilatory rate of 20 breaths per minute, the total respiratory cycle (inspiration + exhalation) = 3 seconds. The inspiratory time (calculated above) is 0.6 seconds, therefore, the exhalation time is 3 – 0.6 = 2.4 seconds, and the inspiratory/expiration ratio (I:E) is approximately

1 : 3. Now let us say that you decided to increase the flow on the ventilator in this patient from 50 L/min to 90 L/min. Go through the same calculations above and you should come up with an inspiratory time of 0.3 seconds. This would mean that the expiratory time would be 3 – 0.3 = 2.7 and an I:E of approximately 1 : 9. As stated previously, always look at the flow-time

graphs on the ventilators to make sure the exhalation returns to baseline before the next breath begins, thus avoiding the stacking of breaths which will lead to auto-PEEP and hyperinflation.

Now if you decrease the ventilatory rate from 20 to let's say 12, the total respiratory will increase from 3 to 6 seconds, and if you keep the flow the same the I : E will increase significantly and will allow the patient to have ample time for exhalation.

Congestive Heart Failure (CHF):

The principles of mechanical ventilatory support in patients with cardiogenic pulmonary edema are similar to the management of patients with non-cardiogenic pulmonary edema. The major ventilatory strategy in these patients includes decreasing the work of breathing and to ensure adequate oxygenation through the administration of adequate FiO_2 and an optimum of PEEP, which will ensure oxygen delivery to tissues. Decreasing the work of breathing may improve heart function by decreasing myocardial oxygen demand.

Myocardial ischemia: Ventilatory strategies are similar to those used in the management of cardiogenic pulmonary edema.

Neuromuscular Diseases

Examples of these diseases include patients with myasthenia gravis, the various forms of myopathies and dystrophies, and patients with cervical cord injuries. Most of these patients have relatively normal airways and pulmonary parenchyma. These patients need ventilatory support because their neuromuscular functions are inadequate to maintain a satisfactory ventilation and they have a tendency to develop atelectasis because of inefficient cough and poor muscle tones. In these patients maintaining an adequate minute ventilation will ensure a satisfactory carbon dioxide elimination which will maintain a satisfactory acid-base balance, and PEEP is likely to maintain a satisfactory oxygenation with a safe concentration of inspired oxygen. Additional pulmonary toilet measures, such bronchodilators, mucolytic agents, and perhaps the use of cough-assist devices may be helpful when one is preparing weaning and liberation from mechanical ventilation in these patients.

Classification of Modes of Positive Pressure Ventilation (PPV)

The next things that you often hear about in the intensive care units are terms such as CMV, AC, SIMV, etc… what do these terms mean?

As we have already discussed, Positive Pressure Ventilation (PPV) is accomplished with a volume or a pressure. You hear about volume-cycled ventilation or time-cycled pressure limited ventilation. This cycling designation refers to the parameter that determines the end of the inspiratory phase, but what about initiation of inspiration? What initiates inspiration? This is described by discussing the various modes of ventilation. The mode of ventilation is what initiates inspiration. There are different modes of PPV. Next, we will discuss the common modes of positive pressure ventilation and their advantages and disadvantages.

Controlled Mechanical Ventilation (CMV)

In this mode, all breaths are mechanically delivered by application of positive pressure to the airway. No spontaneous breaths are allowed and the patient is not able to initiate any additional ventilatory breaths between the set numbers of controlled breaths (see Figure 10). This mode of ventilation is no longer used in the intensive care unit because of the availability of other more desirable modes of ventilation. You may still see it used in the operating room while the patient is under anesthesia.

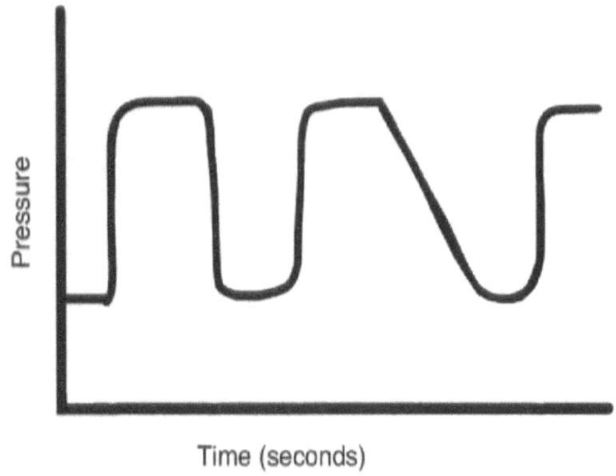

Figure 10 Controlled Mechanical Ventilation

Assist-Controlled Ventilation (AC)

Typically delivered with volume-cycled ventilation. A preset tidal volume is delivered at a preset rate. In addition, each time the patient initiates a breath with a negative inspiratory effort, reaching or exceeding a set threshold (usually a drop in pressure or flow which is referred to as triggering), the ventilator delivers an additional preset *full ventilatory breath* (see Figure 11). Therefore, the patient can increase the ventilatory rate and the ventilatory support on demand. Because each breath that is triggered by and delivered to the patient is a full ventilator breath, weaning is not possible in the AC mode. Therefore, if you are planning on weaning the patient off the ventilator you have to switch to SIMV mode, which will be discussed next.

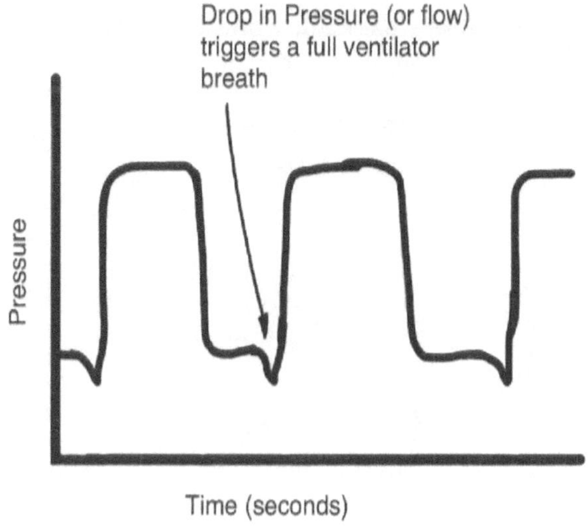

Figure 11 Assist Controlled Mode

Synchronized Intermittent Mandatory Ventilation (SIMV)

Delivers a preset tidal volume at a preset number of times each minute. In addition to these preset ventilator breaths, the patient may access the conditioned gas for a spontaneous breath as frequently and with whatever tidal volume the patient generates (see Figure 12 below). The use of synchronization to deliver a ventilator breath allows for enhanced patient-ventilator interaction and patient-ventilator synchrony. This mode of ventilation may be combined with additional ventilatory modalities such as pressure support ventilation, which is reviewed later in this booklet.

The advantage of SIMV is that it allows the patient to assume a portion of the ventilatory requirement. Negative inspiratory pressure is generated by the patient's spontaneous breaths, leading to increased venous return to the right side of the heart, which in turn improves cardiac output.

During patient generated breaths, there is an additional work burden on the patient. Therefore, SIMV is usually associated with greater work of breathing compared to the **AC** ventilation, and it is less frequently used as an initial ventilator mode in patients admitted to the intensive care unit in acute respiratory failure. However, the extra work generated by the patient for the spontaneous breaths can be minimized by adding a level of pressure support.

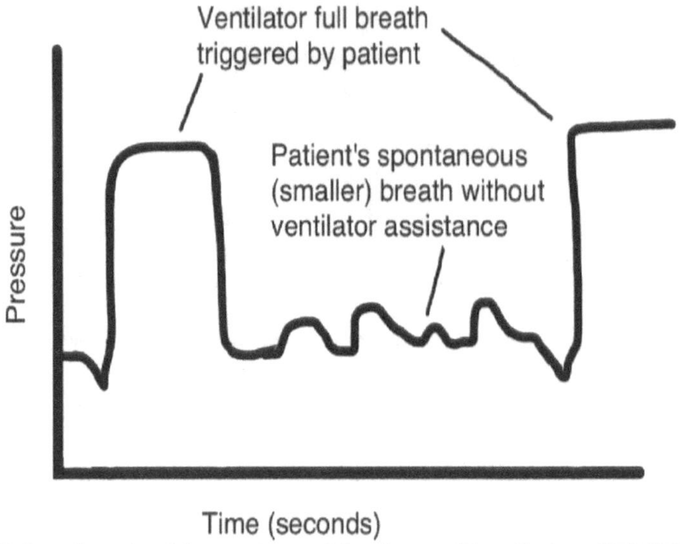

Figure 12 Synchronized Intermittent Mandatory Ventilation (SIMV)

Pressure Support Ventilation (PSV)

This is a form of Positive Pressure Ventilation designed to provide and assist the patient with his/her spontaneous breaths while on PPV in the SIMV mode.

This inspiratory assistance is provided to help the patient overcome the resistance and work of breathing that is necessary to overcome the resistance imposed by the endotracheal tube, the inspiratory valves of the ventilator (if any), and other mechanical aspects of ventilatory support.

With PSV a set amount of pressure support that is applied augments each patient-generated breath. As soon as the patient triggers the ventilator, the set pressure reaches the set limit (example 10 cmH_2O), and it stays there for up to 75% of the duration of inspiration, and then the pressure is withdrawn for the remainder of the inspiratory phase. This will augment the patient's own spontaneous tidal breaths as shown in the Figure 13 below:

The level of pressure support that is necessary to overcome the resistance of the endotracheal tube depends on the size of the tube. The smaller the tube, the higher the level of PS that is needed. It also helps the patient overcome some of the excess work of breathing imposed by the primary disease process. The patient controls the respiratory rate, duration of inspiration, gas flow rate and the tidal volume. PSV may be initiated at 5 cmH_2O and increased by 5 cm H_2O increments to maintain a desired patient's spontaneous tidal volume.

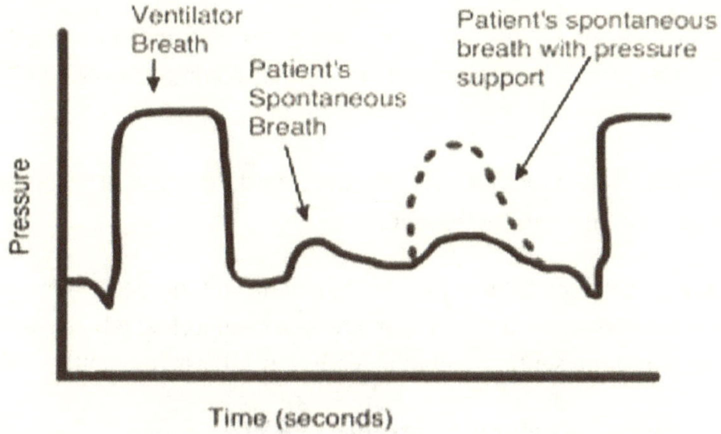

Figure 13 Pressure Support Ventilation

Another guideline for the level of PS based on the size of the Endotracheal Tube (ETT) is as follows:

ETT SIZe	PS (CMH2O)
≤ 3.5	8
4 – 4.5	8
≥ 5	6

As mentioned previously, PSV may also be coupled with SIMV. When PSV is used with SIMV, it augments the patient's spontaneous breaths without any effects on the preset intermittent mechanical ventilator breath. If the patient does not have any respiratory effort, there will not be any ventilatory support, if PSV alone is utilized. A backup ventilation setting is, therefore, required in case of apnea. One caveat of PSV is that in the presence of a bronchopleural fistula or an endotracheal tube cuff leak, there might be interference with appropriate cycling with PSV since flow is accelerated to offset pressure loss due to escaping gas.

Volume Support Ventilation (VSV)

This is simply an automatically regulated pressure support mode. The patient must trigger every breath as in PSV, and therefore, the patient's respiratory drive must be intact and regular to be placed in VSV.

The patient controls his/her own respiratory rate and inspiratory time, as in PSV. However, in VSV the operator sets a tidal volume instead of a pressure support level.

The ventilator then automatically sets and adjusts the pressure support level to maintain the minimum set tidal volume.

If the patient develops fatigue and his/her tidal volume decreases below the set limit, the entilator increases the pressure support level just enough to ensure the minimum set tidal volume. VSV is used less frequently than PSV.

Pressure Regulated Volume Controlled (PRVC):

This is an automatically regulated pressure *controlled mode*. This means that its general principles is similar to an assist-control mode of ventilation.

The tidal volume is preset instead of a pressure level, as in pressure control ventilation (PCV). If the patient's compliance changes, the tidal volume would vary only slightly. However, on the next breath, the ventilator would automatically adjust the pressure level in the proper direction to maintain the target tidal volume. The ventilator maintains a constant airway pressure throughout the entire inspiratory time, and flow is in a variable decelerating profile.

In the initial part of the breath, there is a high flow of gas that allows for immediate attainment and control of PIP and this enhances patient comfort. The flow then decelerates based on the actual physiology of the breath while maintaining a constant airway pressure.

PRVC is **an** assist-controlled mode, so the patient will be ventilated at the set frequency even if the patient has apnea. If the patient's breathing is above the set frequency, each breath is a machine breath at the pressure necessary to maintain the preset tidal volume. Because PRVC is somewhat similar to assist-controlled, it is set and ordered just like the traditional assist-controlled mode of ventilation. Also remember that you will not be able to wean the patient off the ventilator in this mode.

How Does PRVC Work?

Because the ventilator does not know the level of pressure that will be necessary to deliver the preset tidal volume, the first breath in PRVC is a test breath at 10 cmH_2O. The ventilator measures the volume delivered at that particular pressure and calculates the system compliance. The pressure required to deliver this set tidal volume is then determined and the next three breaths ramp up at 75% of the calculated pressure. Therefore, the set tidal volume will be delivered after 4 to 5 breaths. With each breath after this, the ventilator compares the set tidal volume to the actual inspired tidal volume. If the actual and inspired tidal volumes fluctuate, the ventilator will automatically adjust the pressure level up or down on the following breath to maintain a consistent tidal volume. This is all done safely within limits that are manually set.

The ventilator will not adjust the pressure level more than 3 cm from one breath to the next, and the ventilator will not adjust the pressure level higher than 5 cm below the upper pressure limit. If the patient is disconnected from the ventilator, or if the upper pressure limit is reached and less than half of the set tidal volume is delivered, the sequence begins again.

Auto-Mode

Auto-mode is a feature that if the patient triggers two consecutive breathing efforts, it will shift the ventilator from a controlled mode to a support mode. If the patient cannot maintain spontaneous breathing, the ventilator will shift back to the controlled mode after 12 seconds for adults, 8 seconds for pediatric patients, and 5 seconds for neonatal patients.

PRVC/Volume Support

At the second patient triggered breath, the ventilator delivers one more PRVC breath. The breath will be a volume support breath with a pressure level equal to the last PRVC breath. Each breath has to be triggered by the patient, and the pressure support will vary

with each breath. The same principles would apply to volume controlled/volume support and pressure controlled/pressure support.

Airway Pressure Release Ventilation (APRV)

APRV is similar to the application of high CPAP, but with regular intermittent release of airway pressure. It may be used in patients with hypoxemic respiratory failure who need optimization of lung volume. However, APRV is generally reserved for patients with ARDS. By using a sustained airway pressure, collapsed alveoli are recruited, adequate lung volume is achieved, and gas diffusion and collateral ventilation are augmented.

APRV may be considered in patients who are candidates for high frequency ventilation. It may also be considered in patients who are ready to transition from high HFOV to conventional ventilation, particularly if the aim is to avoid muscle relaxants. APRV may be looked at as an inverse ratio ventilation, but the difference is that the patient is allowed to breath spontaneously, thus decreasing the need for sedation and minimizing the use of muscle relaxants. By allowing the patient to breath spontaneously, cardiac filling/output may be maintained and/or augmented. These are some of theoretical advantages of APRV.

The presence of a dynamic expiratory valve in some of the newer ventilators allows spontaneous breathing (throughout the respiratory cycle) at high lung volumes: the ventilator cycles from high to low CPAP.

Terminology for APRV

Pressure high (P_{high}): is the preset inspiratory pressure: initial settings should be equal to the mean airway pressure on high frequency ventilation or 3 - 5 higher than the MAP on conventional ventilation.

Time high (T_{high}): the preset time during which the P_{high} is maintained. Is usually set at 6 seconds.

Pressure low (P_{low}): is the release pressure; during this period the high pressure (P_{high}) is released usually to zero, thus the name APRV.

Time low (T_{low}): is the preset length of time the pressure is released or the P_{low} is maintained. You may also look at this as the expiratory time. This may be set at 0.6 seconds.

P_{high} and T_{high}: control and regulate mean airway pressure and lung volume. These 2 parameters affect oxygenation and ventilation. To improve oxygenation: increase P_{high} by 1 - 2 cm H_2O up to 10 cm H_2O. If no improvement is noted and P_{high} is > 30 cm H_2O, increase T_{high} by 0.5 – 1.0 second increments. Now remember that the cycle rate = 60/ T_{high} + T_{low} and generally cycle rates > 12 lessen the recruitment beneficial effects of APRV. It is preferable to have the cycle rate even lower (single digits) in order to maximize recruitment.

Few other terms that are relevant to APRV are:

1. Peak Expiratory Flow Rate (PEFR)
2. End-Expiratory Flow Rate (EEFR)
3. End-Release Lung Volume (ERLV): which is the volume obtained at the end of the release phase.

4. Spontaneous volume: which is the volume achieved by the patient's spontaneous breaths.

Patient Management

To improve oxygenation:

1. Slowly increase P_{high} . If no improvement is noted after increasing P_{high} by 10 cm H_2O (and P_{high} is > 30 cm H_2O), consider slowly increasing T_{high} in 0.5 – 1.0 second increments

2. As you make these adjustments, make sure that the EEFR is at least 25-50% of the PEFR. This is important so that the patient's Functional Residual Capacity (FRC) is maintained.

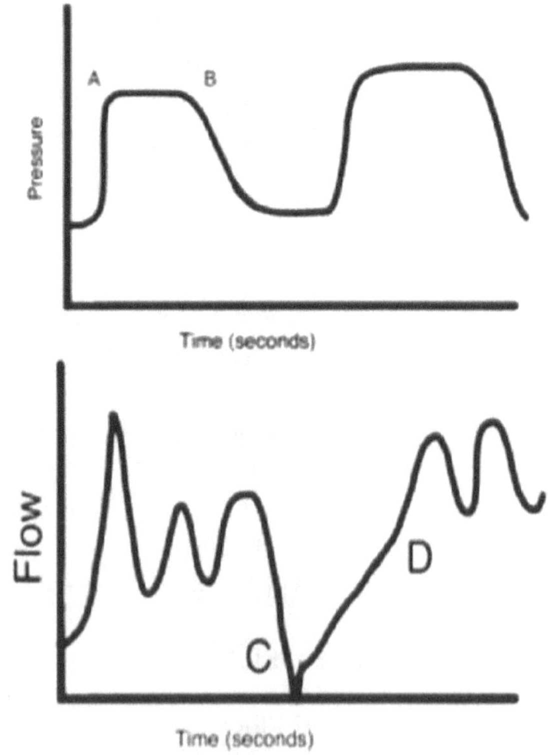

Figure 14 The top graph is the pressure pattern where the high pressure is initiated at point A and maintained until point B, where the pressure is

released. The bottom graph is the flow pattern. As the pressure is released the flow accelerated to point C, which is the peak expiratory flow rate (PEFR), then the flow decelerate to point D which is the End-Expiratory Flow Rate (EEFR). In practice, there is a cursor that you may move from the right to left or vice-versa on the flow graph, until you are at points C (PEFR), and point D (EEFR). You will read from the screen the corresponding flow rate. From these two datas you can calculate the ratio of EEFR/PEFR, which should be 25-50% in order to maintain the FRC.

To Improve Unacceptably High $PaCo_2$

Increase P_{high} by 1 - 2 cm H_2O until it is > 30 cm H_2O. If $PaCO_2$ is still high, you may increase T_{high} by 0.5 – 1.0 second increments. Always make sure that EEFR/PEFR is 25 - 50% by adjusting T_{low}. If the patient's spontaneous tidal volume is low (< 5 ml/kg) adding some level of Pressure Support (PS) may improve ventilation and may help decrease the $PaCO_2$. However, be certain that the total pressure (PIP) does not exceed 35 cm H_2O.

Weaning Patients From APRV (also discussed in the weaning section):

1. Decrease P_{high} by 1 - 2, but increase T_{high} by 0.5 – 1.0 second increments; the goal is to allow the patient to spend more time at P_{high}, which will maximize lung volume.

2. When the P_{high} reaches 15 cm H_2O, and FiO_2 is weaned to < 0.5, you may consider extubation readiness tests.

3. While weaning, keep T_{low} the same. Adjust this parameter only to maintain the EEFR/PEFR between 25 - 50%.

4. If the patient fails, return to the previous settings on the APRV and consider weaning at a later time.

Neurally-Adjusted Ventilatory Assist (NAVA)

Patients receiving conventional mechanical ventilation can be either paralyzed with neuromuscular blockade agents in which case the positive pressure ventilation is controlled entirely by the ventilator and the settings on the ventilator are controlled and adjusted by the operator. Alternatively, the patient may be allowed to breath spontaneously in which case the full ventilatory breaths are synchronized with patient's spontaneous breath or spontaneous breaths are assisted with pressure (pressure support) or volume (volume support) or flow. In this latter case, the ventilator senses a drop in pressure or flow (which are the result of patient's efforts) in order to synchronize a breath with the patient's breath. As we all know that the impulse for initiation of a breath originates in the respiratory centers in the brain stem. These impulses travel via the phrenic nerve to the diaphragm (and intercostals muscles) to stimulates these muscles to contract, which in turn leads to an inspiratory effort that leads to initiation of a breath. Therefore, with the current modality, the ventilator senses the last step in this process and accordingly it delivers a breath.

NAVA is a new modality of ventilatory assist in which the neural impulses generated in the respiratory centers and received by the diaphragm are coupled with ventilation as follows:

Electrical signals are generated in the respiratory centers in the brain stem

- These signals travel to the diaphragm via the phrenic nerve and stimulate the diaphragm to contract and initiate inspiration

- The electrical activities in the diaphragm are detected by special electrodes mounted at the end of a (special) nasogastric that is inserted into the lower part of the esophagus/proximal part of the stomach.

- Electrical signals are transmitted from the special nasogastric tube to the ventilator

- The ventilator equipped with a special module to receive and analyze these signals, converts these signals into a ventilator breath, which assists the patient's spontaneous breath by delivering a calculated pressure

- The ventilator generates a peak inspiratory pressure (PIP) based on the amount of electrical activity generated by the diaphragm

- This PIP translates into a tidal volume for each breath

- PIP is continued until the electrical activity decreases by 45-70% and then the breath is terminated; therefore, the patient determines the PIP and the inspiratory time (Ti) for each breath as well as the respiratory rate (since the patient will receive a breath only if there is a electrical impulse from the brain).

These sequences of events are shown schematically in the diagram below.

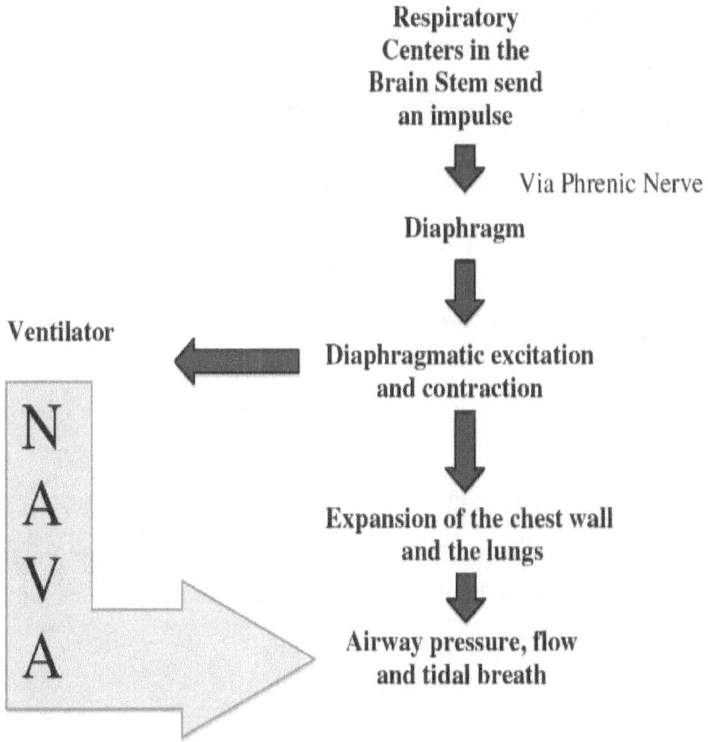

Terminology of NAVA:

Electrical activity of the diaphragm (**Edi**)

Peak Edi: connotes the peak neural inspiratory electrical activity

Edi Min: The tonic (baseline) electrical activity. This electrical activity is believed to play an

important role in preventing de-recruitment of the lungs

Edi trigger: The change (delta) in Edi that is necessary in order to trigger the ventilator to deliver a breath.

NAVA level: a conversion factor that translates the Edi as an electrical impulse to a PIP (cm $H_2O/\mu Volt$)

How is diaphragmatic electrical activity (Edi) measured?

The diagram in the next page illustrates how Edi is measured.

Placing the nasogastric (NG) tube:

- Measure the distance from the xiphoid process to the ear and then to anterior nares.
- The catheter box also contains instructions to determine the length of catheter placement
- dipping the catheter tip in sterile water activates the lubricant present on the tip of the catheter
- Insert the NG tube in the usual fashion to the predetermined length

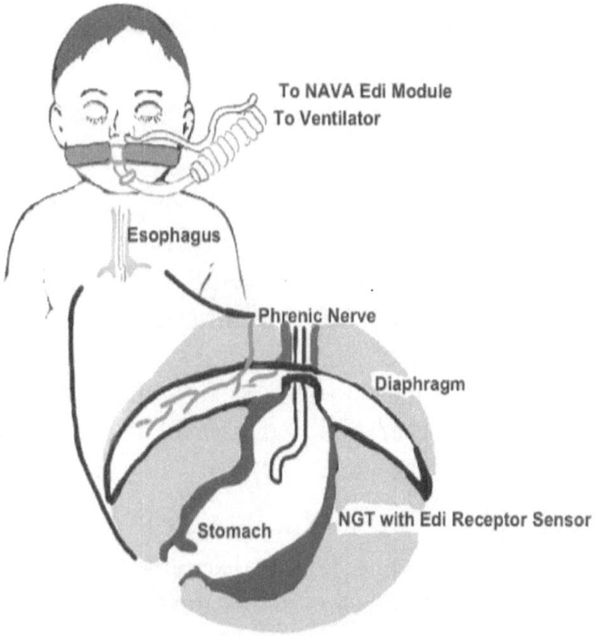

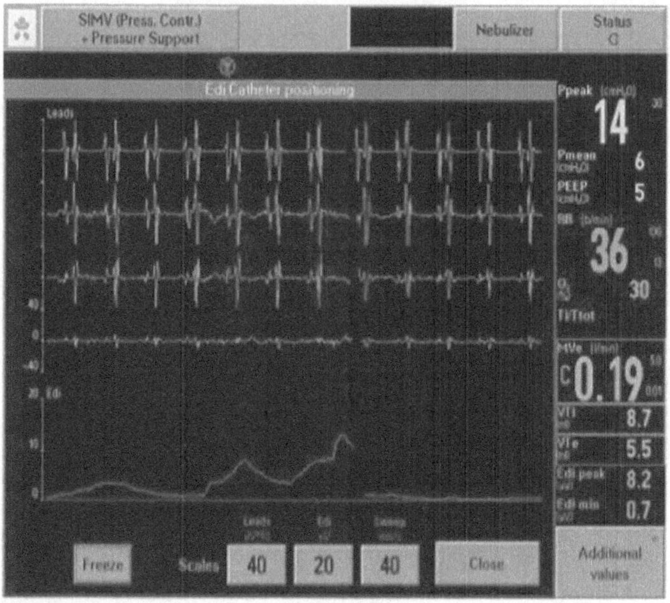

How to set up NAVA?

- If the NAVA module is not already in the ventilator, place it in the ventilator at this time.
- Connect the NG tube to the module at this time
- Position the catheter using the catheter positioning screen on the ventilator screen. The screen will display 3 electrical impulse waveforms from three channels from the tip of the NG tube and an EKG rhythm strip and it will indicate at the bottom of the screen "Nasogastric tube in correctly". This screen will also begin to display the Edi waveform at the bottom of the screen. If the EKG rhythm strip DOES NOT show EKG in the normal sequence (P wave, QRS, and T wave), the catheter is probably is not in a correct position.
- Adjust NAVA level (in cm H_2O per μvolt) to a level that will produce an appropriate PIP that will produce the appropriate tidal volume. On the ventilator screen a new pressure waveform will be superimposed on the current pressure waveform. When the two waveform match, you probably have the appropriate level of NAVA.
- Example: let us say to you set up your Edi level at 2, Edi Peak at 12 and Edi min at 2, and you set the PEEP at 5 cm H_2O. The PIP = NAVA level X (Edi Peak-Edi min) + PEEP
- = 2 (12-2) + 5 = 25 cm H_2O
- Set up appropriate levels of pressure control and pressure support for back up
- Set up the appropriate parameters as follows:
- Go to ventilator mode selection and select NAVA
- Enter the settings including: NAVA level, trigger sensitivity level (0.3 – 0.5 μVolt; remember this the lowest level that initiates a breath), PEEP, FiO_2 , Pressure support parameters (including trigger flow e.g. 5, Inspiratory cycle off e.g. 30%, and pressure support above PEEP e.g. 10 cm H_2O), and
- Back up pressure control parameters: e.g. Pressure control above

PEEP of 10 cm H_2O and back up rate.

– And finally press accept in order to initiate NAVA.

– Adjust alarms as appropriate including upper limit of pressure, minute volume, respiratory rate range, end-expiratory pressure range (e.g. 2–10 cm H_2O) and apnea alarm (e.g. 20 seconds).

Volume Assured Pressure Support Ventilation (VAPS):

This mode of ventilation operates in the Assist/Control, Synchronized Intermittent Mandatory Ventilation, and pressure support modes. On ventilators that have this capability, VAPS is activated by depressing the key labeled **VAPS.** A light should appear above the key to confirm the operation in the VAPS mode.

In the VAPS the ventilator begins each breath as if it is in a pressure supported breath. (please refer to pressure support ventilation for more details). This means that a very rapid initial flow is delivered in order to achieve the preset pressure limit at the airway. As long as the patient flow exceeds the minimal flow, the breath continues to behave like a pressure supported breath i.e. the breath is patient triggered, pressure limited, and flow cycled. If however, the flow returns to the set minimal flow and the desired tidal volume has not been achieved, the set minimal flow persists until the desired tidal volume is reached. If the desired tidal volume is still not reached, volume cycling (instead of flow cycling as in pressure support mode) will take place to deliver the desired tidal volume, thus the term volume assured ventilation.

Advantages & disadvantages of Selected Modes of Mechanical Ventilation

Mode	Advantages	Disadvantages
CMV	Rests muscles of inspiration	No patient-vent interaction; requires use of sedation; potential adverse hemodynamic effects
AC	Patient determines amount of vent support; reduced WOB	Potential adverse hemodynamic effects; may lead to inappropriate hyperventilation
SIMV	Improved patient-vent interaction; less inter- ference with normal cardiovascular function	Increased WOB may be inappropriate unless PS is added
PSV	Patient comfort; improved patient-vent interaction; decreased WOB	Apnea alarm is only back-up; variable effect on patient tolerance
PCV	Allows limitation of PIP; Control of I:E ratio	Potential hyper- or hypo- ventilation with lung resistance/ compliance changes

(WOB = Work of Breathing)

What Do You Do Next If the Patient Continues to be Hypoxemic ?

Let's assume that with a MAP of *25* cmH_2O, a plateau pressure of *35* cmH2O, and a high FiO_2 , the patient continues to be hypoxemic. As indicated previously, you can go to a trial of inverse ratio ventilation (by progressively increasing IT until I:E is reversed) in the pressure controlled mode with decelerating waveform pattern, which is referred to as PC-IRV. It has hypothesized that the decelerating waveform (as opposed to the square waveform) leads to a more uniform distribution of ventilation.

In pressure controlled ventilation with a decelerating waveform, the flow is very rapid at the beginning of inspiration until the preset PIP is reached, then the flow decelerates for the rest of the inspiration.

During the initial rapid flow phase (acceleration phase), the relatively normal alveolar units, with normal resistance and compliance, are inflated (ventilated). Then, during the second phase (the decelerating phase), alveolar units with either increased resistance or altered compliance are slowly ventilated. This leads to a more uniform distribution of ventilation. Refer to Figures 15 and 16.

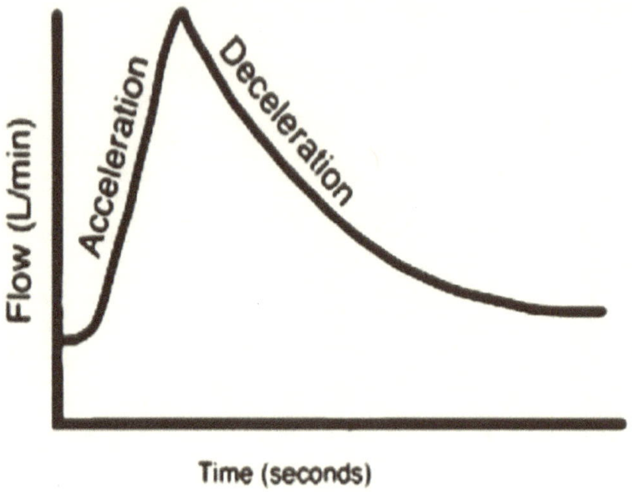

Figure 15

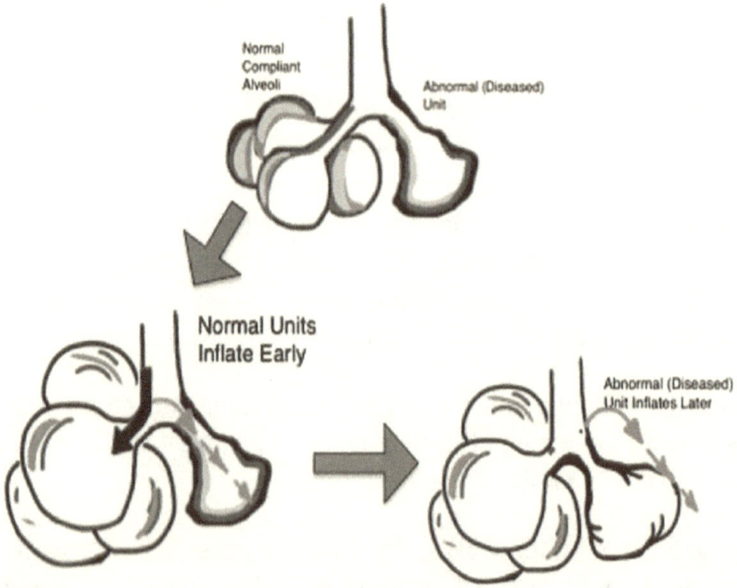

Figure 16

If this strategy does not improve the oxygenation, then you have a number of other options that include, but are not limited to, the following:

1. Prone Ventilation

2. High Frequency Ventilation (HFV)

3. Nitric Oxide (NO)

4. Extra-Corporeal Life Support (ECLS)

PRONE VENTILATION

Sometimes conventional mechanical ventilation with high PEEP may not improve oxygenation or occasionally it may lead to deterioration of oxygenation in patients with significant pulmonary parenchymal disease such as severe ARDS. Two possible mechanisms for the ineffectiveness of PEEP in these settings are:

1. Redistribution of blood flow away from ventilated units = units closer to the anterior (ventral) aspect of the chest, towards units that are less ventilated = units closer to the posterior (dorsal) aspect of the chest.

2. Over-riding of the hypoxic pulmonary vasoconstriction.

One of the interventions that has been found to be useful is *prone position ventilation*, which helps improve oxygenation based on the following putative mechanisms:

- Pulmonary perfusion in the supine position is usually non-homogenous with dorsal dependent lung units receiving most of the blood.

- In the supine position, the tendency for alveolar collapse is also greatest in the dependent dorsal lung units.

- PEEP may redistribute blood flow further away from the upper most ventral lung units (which have higher transpulmonary pressure) towards the dependent dorsal lung units (which have lower transpulmonary pressure) when applied in the supine position.

- It has been postulated that the transpulmonary pressure (alveolar pressure – pleural pressure) is ***more homogenous in the prone***

position, and therefore, the uniform pressure distribution is less likely to be altered by PEEP. This homogenous pressure distribution would lead to uniform expansion of the lungs in the prone position with little redistribution of pulmonary perfusion within the lungs when PEEP is applied. Such a mechanism would contribute to improved gas exchange by improving the ventilation/perfusion (V/Q) ratio in the prone position. However, the mechanism(s) by which prone positioning improve oxygenation is not entirely clear and is probably multifactorial. What complicates matters further is the fact that often other interventions are being done simultaneously in these critically ill patients. Prone positioning should be done in consultation with an experience critical care physician who has adequate resources at her/his disposal. Large randomized trials have not shown an improvement in mortality with prone positioning, however, in most patients some improvement in oxygenation and ventilation is noted. In children with ARDS, Curely, et al showed that prone ventilation improves oxygenation, but does not improve outcome from ARDS (Curely, et al JAMA 2005). Prone ventilation is more likely to improve oxygenation when it is applied early in the course of ARDS.

Technique

1. Turn patient to the lateral position (right or left) paying close attention to O2 saturation, hemodynamics and the various cords and tubes attached to the patient.

2. Turn the patient to full prone position with arms along side and head turned to the right or left.

3. Shoulders and face may be supported with a folded sheet or small blankets.

4. Electrodes for cardiac monitoring may be placed on the patient's back.

5. Intolerance is generally considered present if

a. O_2 saturation drops by > 5% and does not improve

b. BP drops by > 25 mmHg and does not improve

c. Dysrhythmias noted

Early tracheal suctioning should be performed due to mobilization of secretions.

ABG's may be obtained before and at one and four hours after turning patient to prone position.

Non-response may be defined as failing to meet the objectives of: **$FiO_2 \leq 0.6$ with Pa $O_2/FiO_2 > 150$.** (approximately 60% of patients do respond within 2 hours.)

Recruitment Maneuvers:

Because mechanical ventilation preferentially diverts airflow to the non-dependent regions of the lungs, in contrast to the normal physiological pattern where the bases are better aerated, lung collapse is predominantly in the dependent regions of the lungs in most ventilated patients.

Recruitment is a strategy aimed at re-expanding collapsed lung units, and then maintaining high PEEP to prevent subsequent 'de-recruitment'. In order to recruit collapsed lung tissue, sufficient pressure must be imposed to exceed the critical opening pressure of the affected lung. In dependent areas of the lung, the pressures required may exceed 50cm H_2O. Such pressures are *far* in excess of pressures needed to recruit areas of lungs that are not involved with the disease process and in fact may even over-distend these areas of the lungs. A strategy is needed to limit trans-alveolar pressures in the less diseased units of the lungs, but provide sustained high pressures in the diseased units of the lungs sufficient to cause recruitment of these collapsed units.

Ideal patients for recruitment maneuvers are patients with putative ARDS in the early phase of the disease prior the onset of the fibro-proliferative stage and who are poorly oxygenated on a high FiO_2. Pre-existing focal lung disease that may predispose to barotrauma should be regarded as a relative contra-indication to this maneuver. Patients with "secondary" ARDS; e.g. following sepsis are thought to be more likely to respond favorably to recruitment maneuvers than patients with "primary" lung disease and acute lung injury.

The technique:

Sustained inflation of 40 cm H_2O for 40 - 90 seconds as tolerated by monitoring the BP and HR. This can be done by raising the PEEP from its current level of 40 cm H_2O and maintaining for 45 seconds while monitoring the patient. Then reinstitute the ventilation as before. During the period of sustained inflation the ventilatory rate should be set at close to zero so that it is not interrupted by ventilatory breaths.

High Frequency Ventilation (HFV)

HFV is defined as ventilation at a rate > 150 bpm with a tidal volume less than the dead space. There are various types of HFV, which vary in their rates, tidal volume and the system used to deliver gas. Three distinct modes are:

1. High Frequency Positive Pressure Ventilation (HFPPV)
2. High Frequency Jet Ventilation (HFJV)
3. High Frequency Oscillatory Ventilation (HFOV)

The following table shows their features:

Mode	Rate	Volume	Tidal Exhalation	Gas Entrainment
HFPPV	60-100	3-5ml	Passive	None
HFJV	100-150	2-5ml	Passive	Yes
HFOV	Up to 2400	<3ml	Active	Yes

HFOV is the most commonly used type of ventilation and is further discussed below. In adults, ultra-high frequency jet ventilation may also be used, and is described at a later point.

High Frequency Oscillatorv Ventilation (HFOV)

Oscillations are generated by a to-and-fro movement of a piston. On inspiration a column of gas is pushed into the airway and during exhalation gas is drawn out of the airway so that both inspiration and expiration are active. With HFOV, oxygenation is a function of FiO_2, and mean airway pressure (MAP), which is also called continuous distending pressure (CDP).

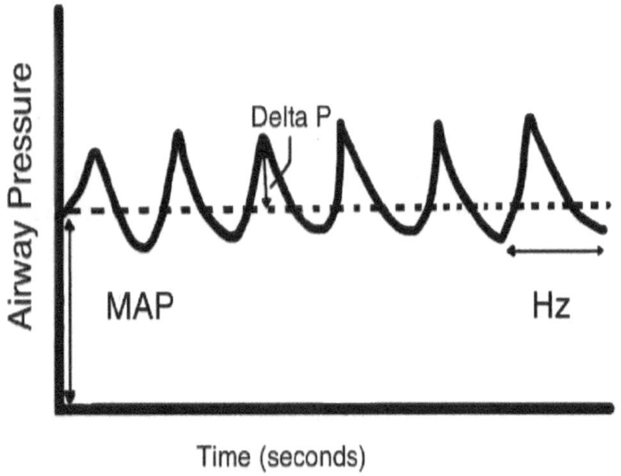

Figure 17 Shows the pattern of ventilation during high frequency ventilation.

The vatrious parameters including mean airway pressure (MAP), pressure amplitude (delta P) and frequency (Hz) are shown

Ventilation is a function of the ventilatory frequency and pressure amplitude (delta P). The inspiratory time is usually set at 0.33 of total cycle. The schematic diagram below (**Figure 17**) shows the pattern of ventilation and various parameters during HFOV. As you can see, the pressure amplitude (delta P) oscillates around the MAP at the preset ventilatory frequency expressed in Hertz (Hz); one Hz = 60 cycles/minute or 60 bpm.

Criteria to Initiate HFOV in Children (does not include neonates)

1. Alveolar-Arterial O_2 gradient > 300 on FiO_2 1.0
2. PEEP ≥ 10 cmH_20
3. MAP ≥ 15 - 18 or PIP ≥ 35
4. Oxygenation Index (OI) > 13 in two ABG's within one
5. hour period (OI = MAP x FiO_2 x 100 ÷ Pa02)

Relative Contraindications

6. Obstructive lung disease

7. Elevation of ICP

8. Hypotension that is poorly responsive to fluid and pressors/inotropes

9. Passive pulmonary blood flow
    j. Modified Fontan procedure
    k. Glenn anastomosis

Where to Start with HFOV

Suction the patient well. Give the patient inspiratory breath at 35 cmH_2O, sustained for 20 to 30 seconds.

MAP: Generally you need to start at a MAP that is 20-30% higher than the MAP on the conventional ventilator prior to switching to HFOV, due to dissipation of delivered pressure along the airway to the alveoli. Occasionally you may have to start even higher and as the oxygenation improves and stabilizes, then gradually decrease the MAP (or CDP).

Lung volume optimization (an increase in PaO_2 enabling you to wean FiO_2

may be attempted immediately after initiation of HFOV, as follows:

Increase MAP (or CDP) repeatedly, in increments of 1 - 2 cm H_2O, every few minutes until adequate oxygenation is achieved ($PaO_2 > 60$ or O_2 saturation of > 90%**).** Keep MAP at the optimal value until you are able to decrease $FiO_2 \leq 0.6$. You may lower the MAP in the same stepwise fashion during weaning.

Always evaluate for hyperinflation (flattening of the diaphragm) by obtaining a chest radiograph within a few hours after instituting HFOV, and every six hours until the patient is stable. If signs of lung over-inflation are present (flattened diaphragm below the **9th** posterior rib), decrease MAP/CDP by **2** cmH_2O and re-evaluate.

Other Parameters

Inspiratory Time (IT) may be adjusted between **0.33** - **0.55,** but is generally kept fixed at **0.33** which is a **1 :2** I:E ratio.

Start ΔP at **10-15** cmH_2O higher than PIP on CMV. The minimum level is **30** cmH_2O; the maximum level is **90** cmH_2O. Watch chest movement to assure adequate chest vibration. Increase ΔP by **5** cmH_2O increments. If maximum ΔP is reached and $PaCO_2$ is still high, decrease frequency in order to decrease $PaCO_2$.

Frequency (Hz):	2- 5 kg BW	10-12 Hz
	5- 10 kg BW	8-10 Hz
	10 -20 kg BW	6-8 Hz
	20 - 25kg BW	5-7 Hz
	25 -45 kg BW	4-6 Hz

Obtain ABG's 20 minutes after the patient has been stable on HFOV. HFOV is used on pediatric patients up to 35-45 kg in body weight.

Technical issues

Currently in the United States, there are two high frequency ventilation devices both manufactured by Sensormedic: 3100 A and 3100B. The 3100 A should be used primarily for children up to 35 kg, although on occasion it may be used for children who slightly heavier. However, the 3100 B is for older children and adults and should not be used for children who weigh less than 35 kg.

High Frequency Ventilation in Adults

In adults HFOV may be used using 3100 B oscillator or the jet ventilator. High frequency jet ventilation (HFJV) delivers small tidal volume which is equal to or less than the dead space at a frequency of 50-100 bpm. This is now referred to as conventional high frequency jet ventilation because more recently, ultra-high frequency jet ventilation (UHFJV) has been introduced which can deliver up to 600 bpm. UHFJV is used for patients 14 years of age and older. Below are some of the practical aspects that you need to know about UHFJV:

1. The Adult Star 1010 is the UHFJV that is most frequently used.

2. You do not need to change the endotracheal tube (ETT) when switching the patient from CMV to UHFJV. Instead, an adapter called proximal monitoring adapter (PMA) is connected to the endotracheal tube (in fact this adapter actually replaces the native endotracheal tube adapter). The PMA is connected to FiO_2, pressure, and temperature monitors (see Figure 13).

3. The other end of the PMA connects to the jet T-piece connection assembly which, in turn, is connected to the ventilator (see Figure 18 below).

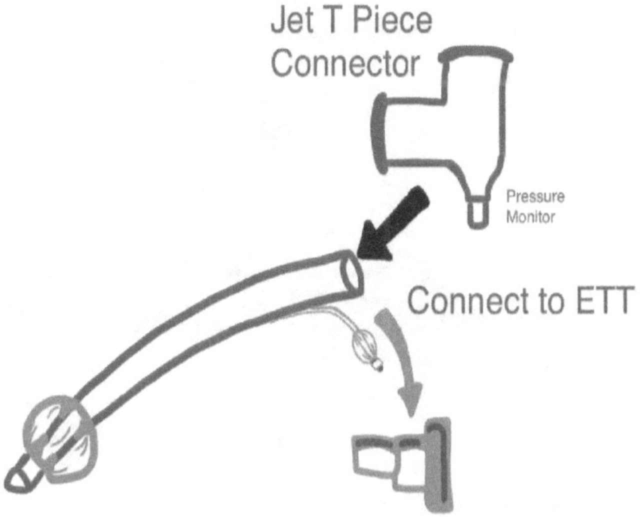

Figure 18

As you can see in Figure 19 below, pressurized gas is received from the hospital supply source (at _50_ psi). The gas then divides into: divides into:

a. Primary Source = Jet Flow = Pulsed Gas

b. Secondary Source = Secondary Flow = Low Pressure Flow

Open exhalation limb (no exhalation valve)

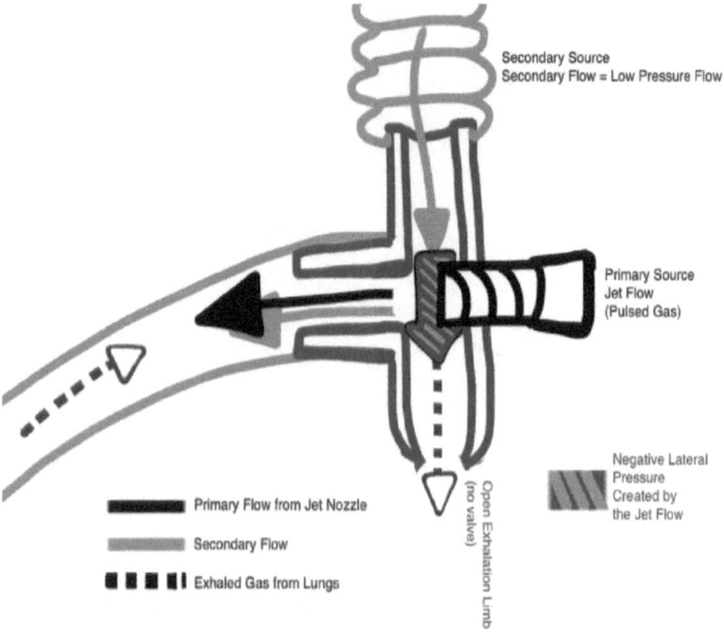

Figure 19: The gas flow patterns during ultra high frequency jet ventilation

In response to a prescribed frequency, inspiratory time, and waveform, the flow from the high-pressure primary (jet) source is interrupted and a high velocity stream of gas is delivered to the patient. Thus, the heart of UHFJV is the mechanism by which high-pressure gas is chopped into small pulses that provide the high frequency breaths.

The secondary flow is entrained (by the negative lateral pressure that is created by the accelerated jet flow) as a continuous flow and delivered to the endotracheal tube.

The Primary (= pulsed = jet) *dry* gas which is 21-100% oxygen, mixes with the humidified and heated 21-100% oxygen gas of the Secondary flow, and the mixture which is now heated and humidified reaches the endotracheal tube which is then delivered to the patient.

Theories of Gas Exchange

There are a number of theories on gas exchange during UHFJV. The basic concept, however, is that the ventilator frequency at which there is the least amount of impedance to gas flow in and out of the lung, is created by this form of ventilatory therapy. In other words, it uses the least amount of force or pressure to get the maximum amount of penetration of volume of gas into the lungs.

Gas exchange is further facilitated due to the fact that the frequency at which air is delivered to the lung approaches the natural resonance or frequency of the adult lung (which is between 4-8 Hz). At this frequency, both oxygenation and ventilation within the lungs are enhanced, and furthermore, the speed of incoming gas pulses (between 240-480 bpm) creates nearly a continuous flow of gas into and out of the lungs.

This latter phenomenon is referred to as convective streaming during jet ventilation and is shown schematically in Figure 20.

Figure 20 Inspiratory and Expiratory Flow diagram

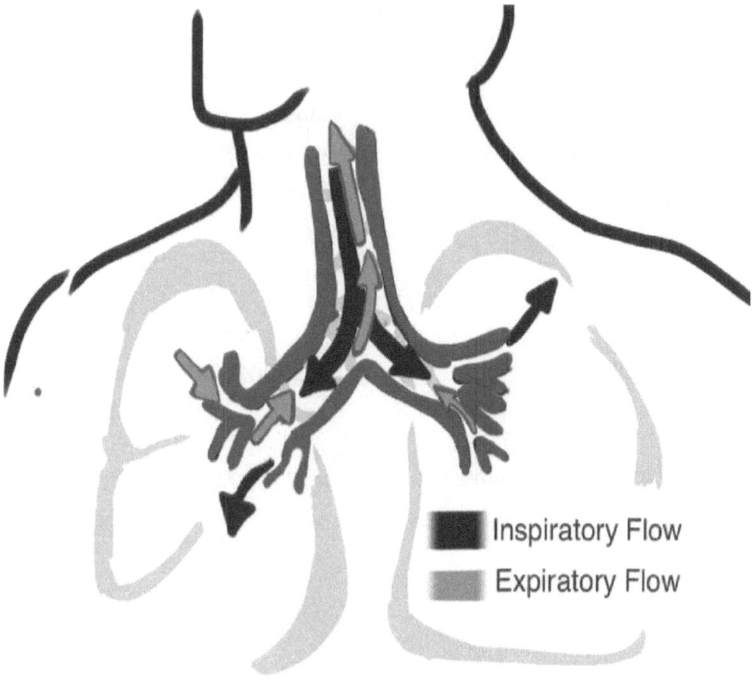

Primary Controls During UHFJV

1. Frequency = Breaths Per Minute and ranges from 1 – 10 Hz

2. Inspiratory Time (IT) = % of respiratory cycle at which gas is delivered.

3. Drive pressure of the primary gas pulse

IT is the most important determinant of Mean Airway Pressure (MAP), although increasing frequency and drive pressure will have a small effect on MAP as well. Increasing the IT will improve oxygen loading by increasing MAP. It is also believed that FRC and alveolar recruitment will increase when IT is increased. Increasing the IT, however, may have an adverse effect on cardiac output if it reaches too high a level.

CO_2 elimination is most dependent upon the drive pressure. Since there is an increase in volume per pulse with increased drive pressure and therefore, a concomitant increase in kinetic energy, the alveoli can be more easily cleansed of CO_2. Increasing the MAP, by increasing the IT has a minimal effect on CO_2. Increasing the frequency of pulsation or breaths per minute while maintaining the same drive pressure and IT, increases the arterial CO2 because the volume per pulse decreases. Decreasing the frequency, therefore, would have the opposite effect and can be utilized when the PaCO2 is elevated.

Control of FiO_2

As mentioned previously, there are two distinct sources of oxygen that combine within the endotracheal tube to provide a final mixture.

The primary (pulsed flow) which is more or less fixed, delivers the following ranges:

1. 21% oxygen (referred to as low)

2. 60% oxygen (referred to as mid)

3. 100% oxygen (referred to as high)

while the secondary flow, which is variable, is capable of delivering any concentration between 21- 100% oxygen.

The primary flow is either diluted by the secondary flow when the oxygen concentration of the primary gas is high, or it is enriched by the secondary flow when the oxygen concentration of the primary gas is low. Since the secondary flow is entrained with each pulse of the primary flow, the

final concentration is measured after having had a chance for adequate mixing, which is approximately 30 seconds.

In practice, one would initially set the primary flow concentration to High (100% oxygen), using a key pad input on the settings and alarms, and the secondary flow concentration to mix by turning the secondary flow blender knob clockwise to the maximum position. The oxygen concentration is then displayed on the monitor panel. After waiting for approximately 30 seconds for equilibration to take place, the blender knob is then turned counter-clockwise until the desired oxygen reading is obtained.

The monitor panel displays, among other parameters, the PIP which you need to know when adjusting the UHFJV settings.

Initial Stabilization of the Patient

Prior to initiation of UHFJV, the patient should be placed on a firm board in order to prevent dissipation of energy. The following are indications for switching a patient from CMV to UHFJV in a patient who has a diagnosis of acute lung injury with normal pulmonary capillary wedge pressure.

1. FiO_2 of > 70% and $Pa0_2$ of < 65 torr

2. PIP > 65 cmH_2O

3. PEEP > 15 cmH_20

Upon transferring the patient from CMV to the Adult Star 1010 for UHFJV, the following initial settings may be used:

1. Frequency: 5Hz

2. Drive Pressure: 32 psi

3. IT: Based on the level of PEEP on CMV prior to switching:

PEEP (CMV)	IT (HFV)
≤ 5	36%
6 - 10	38%
11 - 15	40%
16 - 20	42%
> 20	44%

As you can see, an increase of 2% in IT during UHFJV has the same effect as an increment of 5 cmH_20 of PEEP during CMV.

The patient is then observed at the bedside with pulse oximetry, blood pressure, and other hemodynamic monitoring. Changes to the primary settings, which are the frequency, drive pressure, and IT, are made according to the following observations.

Drive Pressure (DP): You should be able to observe some rocking motion in the lower extremities of the patient. If it appears that there are no movements at all, then the drive pressure should be increased by 2 psi increments until a rocking motion is observed.

Inspiratow Time (IT): If the $Pa0_2$ and/or the O_2 saturation is falling, then IT is increased by 2% at a time until a satisfactory O_2 saturation is established. A few minutes should be allowed to pass between changes.

Frequency (f): Initially, no changes should be made until after obtaining the first arterial blood gas.

Nitric Oxide (NO)

NO is a simple molecule produced from the amino acid arginine and is found in a variety of tissues in the body. When given by inhalation, it is a selective pulmonary vasodilator (by causing smooth muscle relaxation).

NO (when inhaled) will go only to areas of the lungs with relatively normal terminal bronchioles and alveoli. NO causes vasodilation of the pulmonary vasculature only in areas which are in contact with these relatively normal alveoli. In contrast, in areas where the terminal bronchioles

and alveoli are affected by the primary pulmonary process, there is accumulation of inflammatory debris and fluid. This precludes the inhaled NO from reaching the pulmonary vasculature. The end result is matching of ventilation with perfusion. This leads to improvement in the ventilation/

perfusion (V/Q) ratio, which in turn, leads to an improvement in oxygenation.

The source of NO is connected to the ventilator circuit (either conventional or HFV) and delivered along with O_2 at the appropriate dose. NO plus O_2 may produce NO_2 (Nitric dioxide) which is very toxic. The level of NO_2 is continuously monitored on the same panel that displays the NO dose. Thus, levels of both NO and NO2 are known before the inspired gas mixture reaches the endotracheal tube.

NO immediately binds to hemoglobin (as soon as it reaches the circulation) to form methemoglobin, which is toxic in high concentration. Therefore, monitoring of methemoglobin is necessary. Methemoglobin is broken down to nitrates and nitrites that are renally excreted.

The dose of NO is expressed in parts per million (PPM). One PPM is approximately 1 mg/liter. Generally, you may start NO at 5 -10 PPM and gradually increase the dose and titrate to effect. The dose range is quite wide but falls within 5 - 80 PPM. However, most clinicians start NO at 20 PPM and adjust the dose thereafter, based on the patient's underlying disease and therapeutic goals.

NO may be of benefit in patients with ARDS with persistent hypoxemia, however, the beneficial effects may be transient.

No in the Newborn

NO is useful in the treatment of newborns with persistent pulmonary hypertension (PPHN). By reducing the pulmonary vascular resistance (PVR) and pulmonary artery pressure (PAP), shunting across the patent ductus arteriosus is reduced with resultant improvement in pulmonary blood flow. This, in turn, results in improved arterial oxygenation.

Inhaled NO has also become an important adjunctive therapy in the management of patients after repair of congenital cardiac lesions. There appears to be pulmonary endothelial dysfunction induced by cardiopulmonary bypass leading to vascular reactivity. This pulmonary vascular reactivity is responsible for the increase in PVR and PAP that may be seen in the post-operative period. Elevated PVR leads to hypoxemia and/or a decrease in cardiac output, both of which are detrimental to these patients. Inhaled NO has been shown to improve this reactivity and decrease PVR/PAP without compromising systemic perfusion since NO is inactivated within seconds of reaching the vascular system. Examples of cardiac lesions where inhaled NO is of benefit in the postoperative period include Tetralogy of Fallot, atrial ventricular canal defect and right ventricular outflow tract obstruction.

Extra Corporeal Life Support (ECLS)

ECLS (also called ECMO = extracorporeal membrane oxygenation) is probably the last resort (see Figure 18) in patients with persistent hypoxemia and/or hypercarbia with acidemia due to severe respiratory failure or persistent pulmonary hypertension (including pulmonary hypertension in the newborn) secondary to a variety of etiologies when these abnormalities are unresponsive to all other measures of respiratory support previously described.

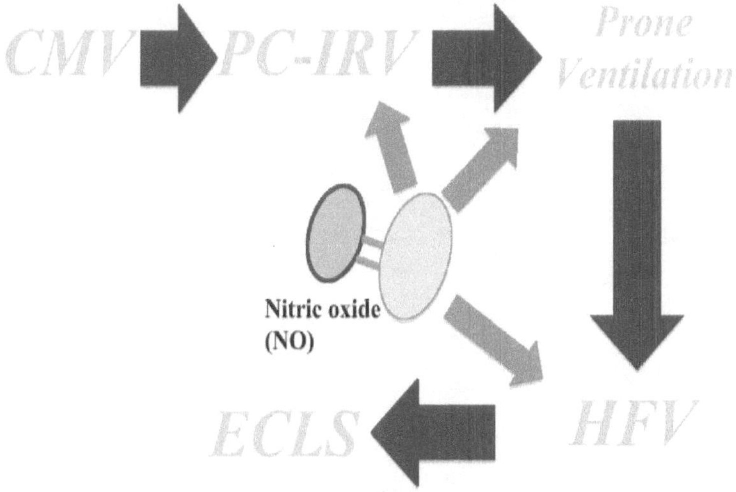

Figure 21

CMV: Conventional Mechanical Ventilation (with high PEEP)

PC-IRV: Pressure Controlled Inverse Ratio Ventilation (with a decelerating waveform)

NO: Nitric Oxide (inhaled)

HFV: High Frequency Ventilation

ECLS: Extra-Corporeal Life Support

ECLS is performed with a roller pump and a veno-arterial (VA) or veno-venous (VV) circuit. During VA ECLS (Figure 22), venous blood is drawn (usually by gravity) using a cannula in the right atrium via the internal jugular vein.

Desaturated blood is pumped through the blood phase of the membrane oxygenator, the gas phase of which is swept with an air/0_2 mixture. Oxygenated blood passes through a heat exchanger, is warmed to body temperature and is then returned to the body via the right common carotid artery. Thus, the lungs are completely bypassed and, at least theoretically, put at rest.

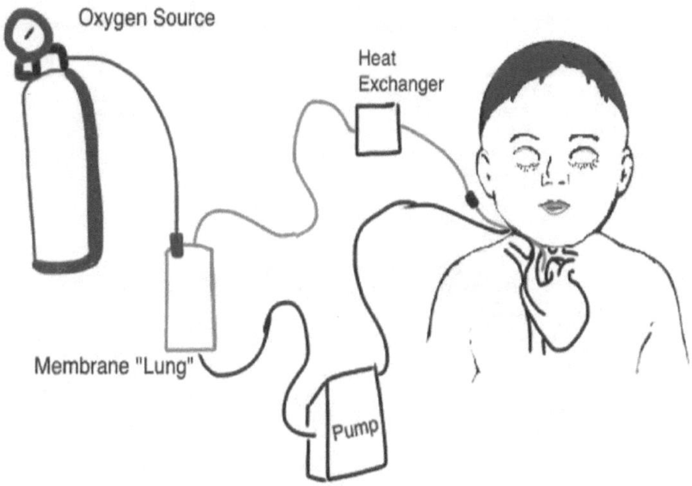

Figure 22 Schematic diagram of an extracorporeal life support circuit.

The rate of flow (of blood from the patient, through the oxygenator, and back to the patient) is usually set at 100 ml/kg body weighdmin. The ventilatory settings usually consist of high PEEP (10-12 cmH_2O) and a ventilatory frequency of 5 bpm while the patient is on ECLS. The algorithm for patients on ECLS is shown in Figure 23.

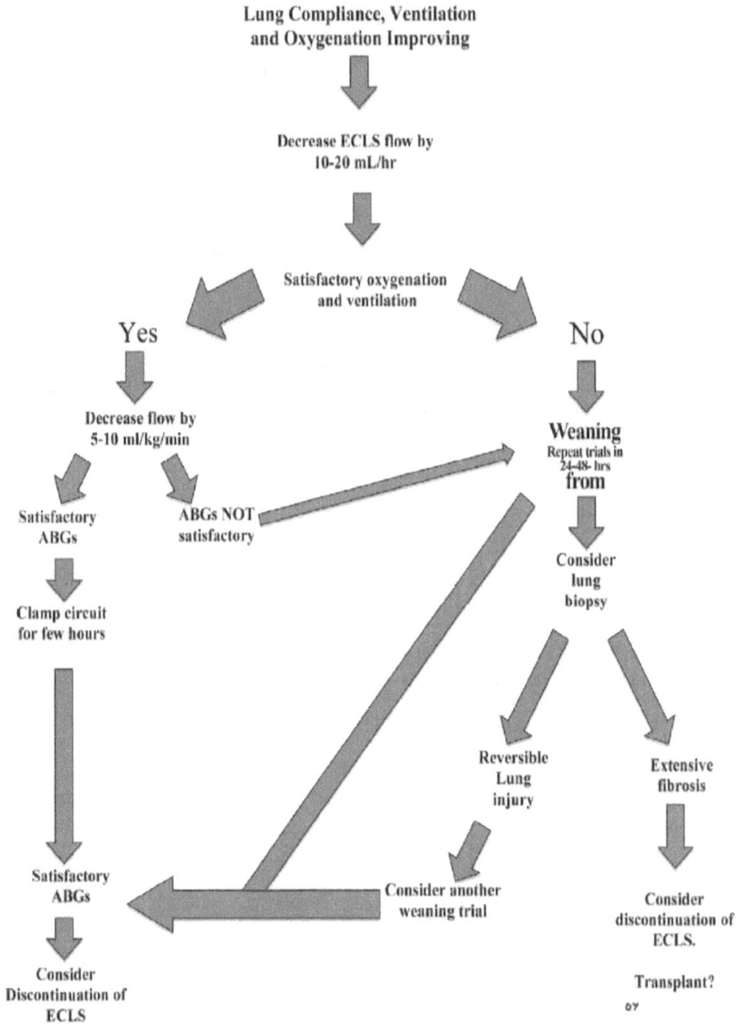
Lung Compliance, Ventilation and Oxygenation Improving
Decrease ECLS flow by 10-20 mL/hr
Satisfactory oxygenation and ventilation
Yes
No
Decrease flow by 5-10 ml/kg/min
Satisfactory ABGs
ABGs NOT satisfactory
Clamp circuit for few hours
Weaning
Repeat trials in 24-48- hrs
from
Consider lung biopsy
Reversible Lung injury
Extensive fibrosis
Satisfactory ABGs
Consider another weaning trial
Consider Discontinuation of ECLS
Consider discontinuation of ECLS.
Transplant?

Weaning from Conventional Mechanical Ventilation in Children

Weaning or liberation from mechanical ventilation is the gradual process during which the level of support provided by the ventilator to the patient is decreased. The patient increasingly assumes the work necessary to generate the tidal breath, and thus, there is an increase in respiratory work commonly referred to as Work of Breathing (WOB). Weaning from mechanical ventilation requires the patient to gradually assume the entire WOB. The controversy regarding the timing of weaning, the pace at which the patient is weaned and ventilator mode selection continues. However, we can make some generalization about the weaning:

- Patients without underlying cardio-respiratory diseases (such as patents with seizures, drug overdose, post-operative care, etc.) usually can be weaned and liberated from mechanical ventilation within a short period of time, usually 24 hours or less.

- Patients with significant underlying cardio-respiratory disease usually require a slow weaning process.

- After cardiac surgery for congenital cardiac defects, prolonged need for mechanical ventilation is unusual. Patients with simpler lesions such as isolated ventricular septal defects, atrial septal defects or uncomplicated tetralogy of Fallot may be weaned and extubated within 24 hours. Patients with more complex lesions may require mechanical ventilation for few days. When these patients require ventilation for longer than 5-7days, a thorough investigation for the presence of an underlying cardiac (residual cardiac defect) or respiratory (such as diaphragmatic paralysis) etiology should be sought.

Timing of Weaning

Appropriate settings to begin weaning include:

1. FiO_2 of 0.5 or less

2. PEEP of 5 cmH_2O or less

3. PIP of 30 cmH_2O or less

4. Ventilatory frequency of 25 bpm or less (or age appropriate ventilatory rate).

Criteria for Weaning

Data on the criteria for weaning in infants and children (compared to adults) is less clear. Maximum negative inspiratory force (NIF) has not been shown to consistently predict weaning in neonates. In older infants and children, a NIF of > 45 cmH_2O and a crying vital capacity (which is not readily available in daily medical practice) > 15 ml/kg body weight predicted successful weaning.

In neonates undergoing repair of congenital cardiac defects, weight gain may be an important determinant of the ability to tolerate weaning. In these patients, cardiopulmonary bypass (CPB) results in fluid accumulation in the interstitium accompanied by a weight gain that may exceed 25% of preoperative weight. Weaning is often possible when weight gain is reduced to 10-20% in excess of pre-operative weight. This can be accomplished by use of diuretics such as Furosamide in the post-operative period after the patient's hemodynamics have stabilized.

Techniques of Weaning:

1. Synchronized Intermittent Mandatory Ventilation (SIMV): Despite lack of definitive data, SIMV weaning has emerged as the standard approach to weaning from conventional mechanical ventilation in infants and children. The gradual reduction in the intermittent mandatory ventilatory (IMV) rate allows the patient to slowly adjust to the increasing workload. The goal is to decrease the IMV rate to 5 or less (in infants and toddlers) or to zero (in older children) while maintaining acceptable blood gases and WOB. The appearance of respiratory distress (tachypnea, retractions), hypoxemia, or hypercarbia are indications to halt further weaning.

2. Pressure Support Ventilation (PSV): PSV requires an effort from the patient and the ability of the ventilator to sense this effort. When a patient (who is breathing spontaneously while on the ventilator) initiates a breath, there is a reduction in airway pressure. The ventilator senses this reduction in airway pressure and immediately delivers a rapid increase in flow until the pre-set pressure (which is the level of pressure support that is set up, say 10 cmH_2O) is achieved. This pressure is maintained until there is a drop in the flow (which is dependent upon the patient's effort) by *25%* at which point inspiration is terminated and expiration begins. This termination of inspiration is totally dependent upon the patient's efforts and ***is not dependent upon volume, pressure or time.***

   The patient retains control of respiratory cycle length, depth, flow characteristics and determines the inspiratory flow, inspiratory time, and frequency. The delivered tidal volume is dependent on: patient efforts, the pre-set pressure support level, and the respiratory system impedence. PSV minimizes the WOB imposed by the endotracheal tube and other mechanical factors in the intubated and mechanically ventilated patient.

   Two methods of weaning during PSV have been advocated:

a. The patient is initially ventilated with a pressure support level that will produce a tidal volume of 8-10 ml/kg body weight. The pressure support level is then gradually decreased to 5 cmH_2O, at which point extubation can be performed if the patient does not exhibit tachypnea and blood gases are satisfactory.

b. SIMV plus pressure support is used in all patients who need to be on mechanical ventilation. The pressure support level is set to achieve a delivered tidal volume of 4-6 ml/kg body weight. As the cardio-respiratory system improves, sedation and paralysis are decreased. The patient increases the number of spontaneous breaths and the SIMV rate is gradually decreased (as above) as the patient's spontaneous efforts increase. The pressure support level is then decreased to maintain a delivered tidal volume of 4-6 ml/kg.

   Patients who exhibit tachypnea, tachycardia and other signs of ineffective gas exchange would be considered to have failed this approach. Extubation should be considered when:

   1) there is a satisfactory PO_2 and PCO_2

   2) the patient is on minimal ventilatory support with SIMV < 5 bpm, PS < 5 cmH_2O, PEEP < 5 cmH_2O, and FiO_2 0.4-0.5

In the largest pediatric study published by Randolph et al, specific weaning protocols was not associated with more successful weaning when compared to no protocol. also there was no difference between pressure support or volume in terms of successful weaning and extubation and the rate of reintubation. What is clear from this study is that children may be weaned and extubated much faster than adults with a median duration of two days. This is a possible explanation for the lack of difference between weaning protocols and no protocols, because the entire process takes a much shorter time compared to adults.

Weaning from Conventional Mechanical Ventilation in Adults

In the adult intensive care unit (ICU), to 20% of mechanically ventilated patients will repeatedly fail attempts at weaning their ventilatory support. Of the intubated patients in the adult ICU, 14% to 22% will require reintubation after being extubated. This increases both hospital cost and mortality rate which can reach 40%. There is not doubt that there is significant room for improvement in this area.

The same methods of weaning discussed above may be used in adults. However, a number of parameters have been studied and have been shown to correlate with successful liberation from conventional mechanical ventilatory support in adults. These parameters include:

1. Parameters that test ventilatory muscle strength:

   - NIF $\geq$ 20 cmH_2O

2. Parameters that test ventilatory mechanics:

   - respiratory rate < 35 bpm and a tidal volume of > 4 mL/kg
   - Vital capacity $\geq$ 10-15 ml/kg
   - Spontaneous tidal volume $\geq$ 5 ml/kg

- Static compliance $\geqq$ 30 ml/cmH_2O

3. Parameters that test ventilatory reserve:

   - Maximum Voluntary Ventilation (MVV)

   (i.e., $\geq$ 2 x minute ventilation with a $PaCO_2$ of 40 torr)

4. Parameters that test minute ventilation (MV):

   - MV < 10 liters /min or

   - $PaCO_2$ of 40 torr or less

   - frequency/tidal volume ratio: < 105 breaths/min/liter

5. Parameters that test dead ventilation:

   - Dead Space (VD) / Tidal Volume (VT) $\leq$ 0.6

It is important to recognize that the above predictors of weaning rely on patient cooperation and effort and have been associated with high false negative predictive rate. Widely accepted clinical parameters associated with failure to wean include: a respiratory rate > 35 bpm, a heart rate > 140 bpm (or an increase or decrease in HR by 20 bpm or more), oxygenation saturation < 90% and the presence of agitation, anxiety or distress.

Weaning from Mechanical Ventilation in Neurosurgical Patients

The approach is slightly different in neurosurgical compared to other patients. There is probably no difference between the various modes of ventilation in these patients. Hyperventilation is often used in these patients in order to decrease cerebral blood flow and intracranial pressure (ICP). This must be used with caution and the arterial carbon dioxide ($PaCO_2$) should not be allowed to drop to a very low level. The $PaCO_2$ is generally kept in the mid-thirties and should definitely not be allowed to fall below 26 torr. Weaning and liberation from mechanical ventilation in these patients is complicated by the fact it is sometimes difficult to assess the level of consciousness and the degree of residual respiratory function. In order to make the correct decision about the timing of weaning and extubation it is important to ask the question of why was the patient intubated. If the reason for intubation was primarily to protect the airway, then the patient should be extubated as soon possible, because prolonged intubation in these patients (particularly adult patients) is associated with a significant risk of ventilator-associated pneumonia. The traditional weaning parameters may not be helpful in these patients. These parameters may still be helpful in patients with ventilatory failure and may be used accordingly. Neurological impairment alone should not be used as the only reason for continuing mechanical ventilation and these patients should be weaned and extubated if their ventilatory functions are adequate.

Non-Invasive Ventilatory Support (NIVS)

NIVS is the preferred method of ventilatory assistance in patients with:

1. Respiratory failure due to neuromuscular disease (NMD)
2. Obstructive Sleep Apnea (OSA)
3. Obesity Hypoventilation Syndrome (OHS)
4. Central Hypoventilation Syndrome (Ondine's Curse)

In addition, NIVS has been used successfully in the following groups of patients in order to avoid tracheal intubation which is associated with nosocomial infection:

1. COPD with exacerbation
2. Hypoxemic respiratory failure of cardiogenic or non-cardiogenic origin
3. As a bridge to transplant in cystic fibrosis and COPD patients

Below are some examples of NIVS:

Negative Pressure Ventilation (NPV)

NPV is used primarily in patients without pulmonary parenchymal disease who require ventilatory support because of neuromuscular disease (NMD). There are limited reports on the use of NPV in patients with pulmonary disease, but for most practical purposes, NPV is utilized mainly for patients with NMD as an intermediate step prior to tracheal intubation and PPV.

The two most frequently used types of NPV are:

1. Cuirass or Turtle Shell: which covers the anterior aspect of the chest like a turtle shell. This device is intended to support a patient's ventilation by alternately applying and releasing external negative pressure over the diaphragm and upper trunk of the patient.

2. Iron Lung: the patient wears a suit which covers the entire body including extremities down to the wrists and ankles. Only the head and neck are exposed.

Principle of Function

Negative pressure is generated around the chest which, in turn, helps with chest expansion, thus augmenting the patient's respiratory effort. This negative pressure (starting at - **8-10** cmH_20) is applied to the chest wall at a specific frequency that constitutes the respiratory rate.

Two other forms of NIVS include *Continuous PositiveAirway Pressure (CPAP) and Bi-Level Positive Airway Pressure (BiPAP).* These are usually administered by a mask of the following type:

- Nasal

- Oral Nasal

- Full Face

These masks are usually secured in place by an elastic head harness. It is crucial for the mask to fit properly in order to minimize air leak and maximize the efficiency of NIVS. It is recommended that different types of masks be evaluated at the bedside and the most appropriate one selected for a patient.

Continuous Positive Airway Pressure (CPAP):

- CPAP is the application of a preset positive pressure throughout the respiratory cycle via a positive pressure ventilator or CPAP device.
- It does not augment patient's ventilation during inspiration.
- It has been shown to improve ventilation and oxygenation in COPD patients and to maintain airway patency in patients with OSA.

It is recommended that you initiate CPAP at 5 cmH_2O and slowly increase the pressure by 2 cmH_20 (every 3-5 minutes) while monitoring the patient's respiratory rate, use of accessory muscles, and pulse oximetry.

Below are the usual CPAP settings for:

COPD	5-8 cmH_20
Pulmonary Edema	Up to 10 cmH_2O

Bi-Level Positive Airway Pressure *(BiPAP)*

- BiPAP is a portable device designed for NIVS.
- BiPAP provides a pressure boost during inspiration, thus augmenting the patient's ventilation.
- BiPAP can be set in the following modes:
  - Spontaneous Mode (similar to Assist-Mode on regular ventilator)
  - Spontaneous/Time (Assist-Controlled)
  - Time Controlled

The latter two modes are used to set a back-up rate to ensure a minimum minute ventilation.

- In patients who tend to hypoventilate during sleep, a spontaneous/time mode is usually used.
- Both inspiratory positive airway pressure (IPAP) and expiratory positive airway pressure (EPAP) can be preset to targeted physiologic points.
- Initial settings, for instance, IPAP of 5 cmH_20 and EPAP of 3 cmH_2O, are slowly increased to a target tidal volume (TV) and to decrease $PaCO_2$ by 5-10 mmHg. If the assist/control mode is utilized, the back-up rate is usually set at 2-4 breaths below the patient's spontaneous respiratory rate to encourage patient's triggering and also facilitate patient-device synchrony. The inspiratory time is usually set at 30%.
- The settings are adjusted to the patient's comfort and the desired TV. With either the assist/control mode or spontaneous mode, the final settings are often:

IPAP:	15 cmH_2O
EPAP:	4 cmH_2O
Frequency:	10 IMV
IT:	0.3

- Supplemental oxygen can be connected to the device tubing using a T-connector. With more recent BiPAP devices, FiO_2 is adjusted in the same fashion as is done on a conventional ventilator.

Helium-Oxygen (Heliox) Mixture

Administration of Heliox:

With laminar flow, the resistance to flow of air is proportionate to ***viscosity*** of a gas. With turbulent flow, the resistance to flow is proportionate to ***density*** of a gas. In healthy human subjects, turbulent flow has been observed in the upper respiratory tract, the larynx and glottis as well as the central airways down to 10th generation of the airways. These portions of the airway are considered density dependent when it comes to airflow. In the setting of airway obstruction these characteristics may be even more pronounced. Remember that when a patient is breathing say 40% oxygen or FiO2 of 0.4, this means that 40% of the gas inhaled is oxygen and the rest of the gas is nitrogen or air. Nitrogen is a more dense gas than helium. In order to decrease the density of the inhaled gas, one could use a mixture of helium and oxygen instead of the usual nitrogen and oxygen.

The use of a low-density gas such as helium may be of benefit to patients with various types of airway obstruction. Use of a less dense gas may significantly reduce the work necessary for ventilation and may also decrease gas trapping.

Clinical Uses of Heliox:

1. Upper Airway obstruction:

A. Pediatric Patient:

1) Laryngotracheobronchitis (viral croup): Heliox may be used in patients with croup to gain time to carry the patient through the period of severe respiratory distress (in order to avoid intubation), until steroids begin to exert their anti-inflammatory and anti-edema effects, or the process of croup gradually resolves. Because the helium-oxygen mixture is less dense than the oxygen-nitrogen mixture, the flow across the narrowed area (subglottic area) will be faster, and the pressure difference required for the same rate of flow would be less for the lower-density gas mixture. This will decrease work of breathing and will lessen fatigue. Clinical improvement in symptoms has been noted with 70 : 30% helium-oxygen mixtures (i.e., 70% helium and 30% oxygen).

2) Post-extubation stridor (subglottic edema): Heliox may be used with the same principles as in croup.

B. Adult Patients:

1) Upper airway narrowing:

a) intraluminal narrowing : mass

b) extrinsic compression

In these cases Heliox may be used while the mass (e.g., tumor) is being treated to reduce its size.

2) Chronic obstructive lung disease (COPD): when an 80:20 helium-oxygen mixture was used in patients with COPD, expiratory flows increased for a given lung volume and there was a reduction in arterial carbon dioxide. Forced residual volume decreased. The authors (Swidwa et al, Chest. 1985) speculated that use of helium, a less dense gas, in these patients could result is less hyperinflation with a change in configuration of the diaphragm and the chest wall. This improves the efficiency of the respiratory muscles, because it places them at a

better mechanical advantage.

C. Both Adults and Pediatrics:

1) Bronchial asthma with acute exacerbation: the helium-oxygen mixture has been shown to be beneficial in patients with status asthmaticus (both adult and pediatric patients). An improvement in pulsus paradoxus, arterial carbon dioxide, dyspnea index and peak flow has been noted with Heliox. The need for tracheal intubation was also decreased in some studies. However, the use of Heliox is adjunctive. It should be used in conjunction with steroids and bronchodilators. Bronchodilators may be administered using the helium-oxygen mixture.

Practical Aspects of Administration of Heliox:

Commercial preparations of a helium-oxygen mixture of 80:20 and 70:30 are available. In patients who do not require an $FiO_2 > 0.30$, a helium-oxygen mixture may be administered directly from the heliox cylinder using a regulator and a flow meter to a ***tightly fitting mask*** It is critical that heliox be delivered through a tight fitting, nonrebreathing oxygen mask (with all one-way valves in place), otherwise the efficacy of heliox may not be appreciable.

A flow rate of 5-10 L/min should be sufficient to provide high flow therapy. If additional oxygen is required to maintain an oxygen saturation of > 90%, low-flow oxygen may be administered via a nasal cannula. When oxygen or airflow meters (as opposed to helium specific flow meters) are used, a flow rate of 5-10 L/min actually provides a flow rate of 9-18 L/min because helium is a less dense gas. To get the actual flow rate a conversion factor must be used. The conversion factor can be calculated by dividing the square root of the gas for which the flow meter is calibrated for by the square root of the density of the helium-oxygen mixture. The desired flow to the patient divided by the conversion factor yields the flow to be dialed in on the meter. Actual flow is calculated by multiplying the correction factor by the flow rate indicated on the flow meter.

Other Practical Aspects of Heliox:

1. While it is commonly stated in textbooks that the ratio of helium to oxygen need to be > 60:40 to gain mechanical advantages, the study by Lu et al does not support this notion and suggests that lower concentrations of helium may still be effective.

2. It appears that the initial beneficial effects of helium-oxygen use begin with its administration, however 20 minutes may be required to demonstrate its full effect. Several studies have shown variable effects over time ranging from 20 minutes to several hours.

3. Helium is several times more expensive than oxygen. Depending on the flow rate, three to six tanks may be needed for every 24 hours of treatment. The cost ranges between $320 to $480 USD/day. There is limited data on the cost-effectiveness of helium therapy.

PEDIATRICS

Where To Start With conventional mechanical ventilation (CMV)?

A. NEONATES

1. FiO_2 of 0.21 to 1.0. Depending on the clinical circumstances, but remember (with all patients, particularly the premature infants) to lower the FiO_2 to 0.6 or less, or the lowest level that would maintain an arterial oxygen saturation of ≥ 90% as soon as possible within 24 hours.

2. PIP of 20 cmH_20 or tidal volume of 5-8 ml/kg. Adjust the levels based on chest expansion, air entry and arterial blood gases.

3. PEEP of 4-5 cmH_2O

4. Ventilatory Rate of 30-40 bpm. Adjust as necessary based on the carbon dioxide levels.

B. TODDLERS

1. FiO_2 of 0.21 to 1.0

2. PIP of mid 20's cmH_2O

3. Tidal volume 5-8 ml/kg body weight

4. PEEP of 5-10 cmH_20

5. Ventilatory Rate of 20-30 bpm

C. OLDER CHILDREN

1. FiO_2 of 0.2 1 to 1.0
2. PIP of high 20's cmH_2O
3. Tidal Volume 5-8 ml/kg body weight
4. PEEP of 5-10 cmH_2O
5. Ventilatory rate of 20 bpm

D. ADOLESCENT

1. FiO_2 of 0.21 to 1.0
2. PIP of high 20's or low 30's cmH_2O
3. Tidal volume 5-8 ml/kg body weight
4. PEEP of 5-10 cmH_20
5. Ventilatory rate of 10-20 bpm

You will need to increase PEEP in order to increase the MAP, as necessary. Remember that PEEP in excess of 10- 12 cmH_20 becomes less and less effective in improving oxygenation.

PEDIATRICS

How to Manipulate CMV in Children?

PROBLEM	*ACTIONS*
Low PaO_2	Increase FiO_2 by 5% increments
	Increase PEEP by 1 –2 (up to 12)
	Increase IT by 0.1 until I:E reversal
High $PaCO_2$	Increase PIP by 2 or
	Increase tidal volume by 1-2 mL/kg
	Increase rate by 5 bpm at a time

ADULTS

Where To Start With CMV?

1. TV: 5-8 ml/kg/body weight
2. FiO_2: 0.21 - 1.0
3. Rate: 10-12 bpm
4. PEEP: 5-8 cmH_2O
5. Use a decelerating inspiratory waveform
6. Flow of 60-80 L/min; 90 L/min for COPD

ADULTS

How to Manipulate CMV in Adults?

PROBLEM	*ACTIONS*
Low PaO_2	1. Increase FiO_2 by 5% increments
	2. Increase PEEP by 1–2 (up to 12) or to Increase MAP up to 25 cm H_2O.
	3. A trial of MAP > 25 cm H_2O by increasing PEEP or IT
	4. Decrease plateau pressure to < 35 cm H_2O by decreasing inspiratory flow, tidal volume or PEEP.
High $PaCO_2$	Increase tidal volume by 1-2 mL/kg
	Increase rate by 2 bpm at a time
	Increase exhalation time by increasing flow

HFOV (PEDIATRICS)

<u>Where To Start?</u>

MAP:	20-30% > MAP on CMV
FiO_2:	1.0
ΔP:	10-15 cmH_2O greater than PIP on CMV, Increase by 5 cmH_2O until good chest vibration is seen.
	Minimum ΔP: 30 cmH_2O
	Maximum ΔP: 90 mH_20

Hz:		
	2-5 kg BW	10-12 Hz
	5-10 kg BW	8-10 Hz
	10-20 kg BW	6-8 Hz
	20-25 kg BW	5-7 Hz
	>25 kg BW	4-6 Hz

HFOV (PEDIATRICS):

How to Manipulate HFOV ?

PROBLEM	*ACTIONS*
Low PaO_2	1. Increase FiO_2 by 5% increments 2. Increase MAP by 1 –2 up to 25 cm H_2O. 3. A trial of MAP > 25 cm H_2O if hemodynamics of the patient tolerate it.
High $PaCO_2$	Increase delta P by 5 cm H_2O Decrease frequency by 2 Hz. If above fail, consider decreasing delta P and Frequency. (minimum frequency 3 Hz).

Review Questions

1. Barotrauma is a recognized complication of positive pressure ventilation. Strategies to minimize this complication have been discussed in this pocket guide. Which of the following ventilatory strategies is expected to be associated with the ***least*** risk of barotrauma:

A. A tidal volume (TV) of 5 ml/kg and a PEEP of 10 cmH_2O

B. A TV of 7 ml/kg and a PEEP of 15 cmH_20

C. A plateau pressure < 35 cmH_2O with a decelerating waveform

D. Peak airway pressure 50 cmH_2O with a square waveform inspiratory flow

E. A TV 10ml/kg and a mean inspiratory flow of 60L/min.

2. Regional lung over-distention at end-inspiration rarely occurs during mechanical ventilation in which of the following setting:

A. Diffuse idiopathic pulmonary fibrosis

B. Acute Respiratory Distress Syndrome

C. Acute exacerbation of Chronic Obstructive Pulmonary Disease (COPD)

D. Auto-PEEP of 15 cm H_20 without bronchospasm (emphysema)

E. Acute bronchospasm with hyperinflation

3. When a patient is receiving conventional positive pressure ventilation at a specific fixed tidal volume, which of the following end-point will result as the conditions change?

A. A uniform expansion of all lung units based on the plateau pressure.

B. A constant plateau pressure in spite of changing respiratory rate.

C. A constant end-inspiratory lung volume in spite of varying airway resistance.

D. A constant increase in intrathoracic pressure despite changes in lung compliance

E. None of the above

4. A 1-year-old boy with ARDS is being assisted with pressure limited ventilation with an inspiratory time of 1 second, SIMV 20 bpm, PIP 30 cmH_2O, and PEEP 8 cmH_2O. The chest radiograph has shown significant improvement over the past 24 hours, and the FiO_2 has been weaned from 0.7 to 0.45. Failure to decrease the inspiratory time may result in all of the following ***except:***

   A. Decreased venous return

   B. Decreased physiologic dead space

   C. Auto-PEEP

   D. Pneumomediastinum

5. Modifications of ventilator circuits for pediatric mechanical ventilation, in order to substantially reduce the system compliance, include all of the following except:

   A. Small diameter circuit tubing

   B. Rigid tubing with the inspiratory circuit as short as possible

   C. Decreasing humidifier size

   D. Positioning of the exhalation valve as far as possible from the airway opening

   E. Maintaining humidifier fluid level

6. A 6-month-old infant with pneumonia (weight 6 kg) is being ventilated: PIP 32 cmH_2O, rate 35 bpm, PEEP 6 cmH_2O, and FiO_2 0.6. The inspiratory time is set at 0.5 seconds and the flow rate is 8 liters/min. What is the approximate tidal volume:

   A. 11 ml/kg

B. 5 ml/kg

C. 9 ml/kg

D. 7 mg/kg

E. 7 ml/kg

7. The alveolar air equation (Pa02 = PI02 - PaCO2/R) ***does not make*** which of the following assumptions:

   A. There is no inert gas exchange

   B. There is no difference in inspired and expired gas volume

   C. Normally more Oxygen is consumed than carbon dioxide produced

   D. Normally the amount of Oxygen consumed and carbon dioxide produced is the same

8. During pressure-control inverse ration ventilation (PC-IRV), tidal volume is a function of:

   A. Respiratory system compliance and resistance

   B. Pre-set pressure limit

   C. The ratio of inspiratory time to the total duty cycle

   D. Frequency (breaths per minute)

   E. All of the above

9. In describing pressure support ventilation (PSV), which one of the following options is ***least*** accurate:

   A. The ventilator retains complete control of the cycle length and depth as well as flow characteristics

   B. PSV has been shown to decrease diaphragmatic muscle fatigue in patients who fail conventional weaning attempts

   C. PSV helps compensate for work of breathing due to the endotracheal tube impedance

   D. Patient effort, level of pressure support and the respiratory system impedance determine the tidal volume

10. The figure below represents the capnogram obtained from a patient on SIMV mode, using a ventilator that has a demand valve. The best intervention is:

A. Substitute the neuromuscular blockade with a non-depolarizing agent

B. Calm the patient and reassure him

C. Add a bronchodilator

D. Add 20 cmH_20 of pressure support

E. None of the above

11. A child with acute respiratory failure is breathing oxygen at a concentration of 40% (FiO_2 0.4). The arterial CO_2 and O_2 are 40 torr and 100 torr, respectively. The respiratory quotient is 0.8. The barometric pressure is 747 and the blood gases are obtained when the patient's body temperature was 37°C. What is the alveolar-arterial oxygen (PAO_2- PaO_2) difference (gradient):

A. 330

B. 190

C. 160

D. 130

E. 20

12. Nitric Oxide is synthesized from which of the following:

A. Arginine

B. Glutamic acid

C. Leucine

D. Isoleucine

E. Linoleic acid

13. A 1-day-old infant underwent insertion of an aorticopulmonary shunt measuring 5mm in diameter for an underlying cyanotic congenital heart disease. He has been admitted to the intensive care unit for

postoperative care and is on conventional positive pressure ventilation. A large left to right shunt is noted while he is on the ventilator. Which of the following is most likely to reduce the left to right shunt blood flow:

A. Hydralazine

B. Increasing FiO_2

C. Administration of inhaled nitric oxide

D. Increasing PEEP on the ventilator

E. Increasing arterial pH

14. A 9-month-old infant who was on mechanical ventilation for pneumonia and respiratory failure was extubated this morning. Which of the following is the earliest evidence of inspiratory muscle fatigue after discontinuation of mechanical ventilation:

A. Alternation of abdominal and thoracic breathing every few breaths

B. Primary thoracic inspiratory efforts when supine

C. An increase in respiratory rate

D. An increase in arterial CO_2

E. Abdomen moving inward during inspiration

15. What is the toxic byproduct of the combination of nitric oxide with oxygen:

A. NO

B. Nitric dioxide

C. Nitrous oxide

D. Hemoglobin

E. All of the above

16. A helium-oxygen mixture (Heliox) has been shown to be of benefit in which of the following clinical situations:

A. Croup

B. COPD

C. Asthma

D. Fixed upper airway narrowing

E. All of the above

Review Answers & Justification

1. C When peak airway pressure is allowed to increase to a level beyond that is necessary to maximally distend the lungs, barotrauma and lung injury result.

   Since regional differences in lung resistance and compliance often co-exist, maintaining a constant VT may over-distend areas of the lung that are aerated if the remainder of the lung is collapsed. Similarly maintaining a constant inspiratory flow pattern when regional differences in lung units exist will selectively increase distention of lung units with lower resistant.

2. D Pulmonary conditions associated with decreased compliance such as pulmonary fibrosis and ARDS or increased airway resistance such as bronchial asthma and COPD have the potential for being homogenous. This homogeneity can result in regional over-distention during positive pressure ventilation. Hyperinflation secondary to airway narrowing or collapse such as seen with auto-PEEP increases end-expiratory lung volume but does not result in lung expansion of the hyperinflated lung units until airway pressure exceeds the level of auto-PEEP. Although the work of breathing during spontaneous breathing is increased by auto-PEEP, end-inspiratory lung volumes do not increase.

3. D Changes in intrathoracic pressure correlate highly with changes in lung volume.

   Changes in intrathoracic pressure are independent of lung compliance. An increase in respiratory rate with lung conditions associated with increased expiratory airway resistant will result in dynamic hyperinflation because there is inadequate time for exhalation. Examples are COPD, asthma, and other causes of intrathoracic airway obstruction. Thus, overdistention is possible with a fixed tidal breath or tidal volume. Since regional lung compliance, even in healthy individuals, is different under all conditions, uniform expansion of all lung units by positive pressure ventilation at any setting probably never occurs.

4. B Hyperinflation which is likely to result from inadequate inspiratory time will result in increased dead space.

5. D The exhalation valve is usually kept as close to the airway as possible in order to minimize the circuit volume.

6. A The flow is set at 8liters/min = 8000 ml/min. = 8000ml/60 seconds. The duration of inspiration is 0.5 seconds. Therefore the approximate tidal volume = (8000 X 0.5)/60 = 66 ml or 11 ml/kg.

7. D The amount of O_2 consumed is greater than the amount of CO_2 produced.

8. E

9. A With PSV, length and depth of the respiratory cycle as well as flow characteristics are determined by the patient and the level of preset pressure support.

10. D This capnogram shows irregularities in the exhalation of CO_2 which would be due to irregularities in the pattern of breathing of the patient, most likely due to patient-ventilator asynchrony or patient's fatigue. Adding 20 cmH_2O of pressure support will decrease the work of breathing and is likely to lead to a more consistent tidal volume and ventilatory pattern.

11. D Alveolar-arterial oxygen gradient = ($PA0_2$ - $Pa0_2$)

$PA0_2$ = Alveolar oxygen tension = $PI0_2$ - $PaCO_2/RQ$

$Pa0_2$ = Arterial oxygen tension

$PI0_2$ = (Barometric pressure - Vapor pressure) X Fraction of inspired oxygen (FiO_2)= 747 - 47 = 700 X 0.4 = 280

RQ = Respiratory quotient = 0.8 in this case

Therefore Alveolar oxygen tension

= (700 X 0.4) - 50

= 280 - 50 = 2 3 0

Alveolar - arterial oxygen gradient

= 230 - 100 = 130

You can also find this equation on page 2 of this handbook.

12. A Nitric oxide is synthesized from the amino acid, arginine by the action of the enzyme nitric oxide synthetase.

13. D Systemic to pulmonary shunt is often created in neonates and infants with an underlying cardiac defects in order to improve pulmonary blood flow and oxygenation. Examples are the (modified) Blalock-Taussig shunt which connects the subclavian artery to the pulmonary artery using a synthetic material and aortic to pulmonary window which usually connects the ascending aorta to the pulmonary artery. Conditions that lead to a reduction in pulmonary artery pressure and pulmonary vascular resistance would increase the flow across the shunt with an increase in left to right shunt. Examples include:

    1. Alkalosis
    2. Vasodilators such as hydralazine and nitroprusside
    3. An increase in the concentration of inspired oxygen
    4. Selective pulmonary vasodilators such as Nitric oxide

    Interventions that lead an increase in pulmonary vascular resistance such as increasing PEEP would lead to a reduction in pulmonary blood flow and a reduction in the left to right shunt.

14. C Tachypnea in this infant would be the earliest evidence of inspiratory muscle fatigue.

15. B Nitric dioxide is the toxic byproduct. The rate of formation of this toxic product is dependent duration of contact between oxygen and nitric oxide.

16. E

www.ingramcontent.com/pod-product-compliance
Lightning Source LLC
Chambersburg PA
CBHW020733160726
47993CB00006B/2430
* 9 7 9 8 7 3 7 4 6 0 4 3 3 *